Dietary Responses to Cancer

By

Lynne D M Noble

All rights reserved. No part of this publication may be reproduced, stored in a retrieval system or transmitted in any form or by any means, without prior permission in writing of the author Lynne D M Noble, or as expressly agreed by law, or under terms agreed with the appropriate reprographics right organisation.

You must not circulate this book in any other binding or cover and you must impose the same condition on any acquirer.

Independently published 2023

About the Author

Lynne Noble was born in 1953 in Huddersfield, West Yorkshire. From a very early age, Lynne showed an interest in nutrition and genetics avidly reading any books that she could get her hands on at the time.

Initially, Lynne studied orthopaedics but events led her to work with the elderly mentally infirm. Here, her interest in neurodegenerative disorders and pain syndromes developed.

Lynne undertook rigorous programmes of study, completing her Cert Ed., (FE) BSc (Hons) and Adv. Dip Education simultaneously before moving onto her M.Ed.

From there she took further demanding programmes in Human Nutrition, Pharmacology, Neuroscience, Genetics and Immunology. During this time, she was given many prestigious awards for her academic work. It was noted then that Lynne was not afraid of tackling difficult subjects.

She began her law degree but ill health prevented her from pursuing this. However, in this time, she moved from being a foster parent to adoptive parent.

She has been instrumental in setting up projects in the community for disadvantaged groups.

She is a member of the Guild of Health Writers.

Now retired, she lives with her husband in a historic Georgian riverside town in the West Midlands. She enjoys gardening, watching her husband bowling and researching.

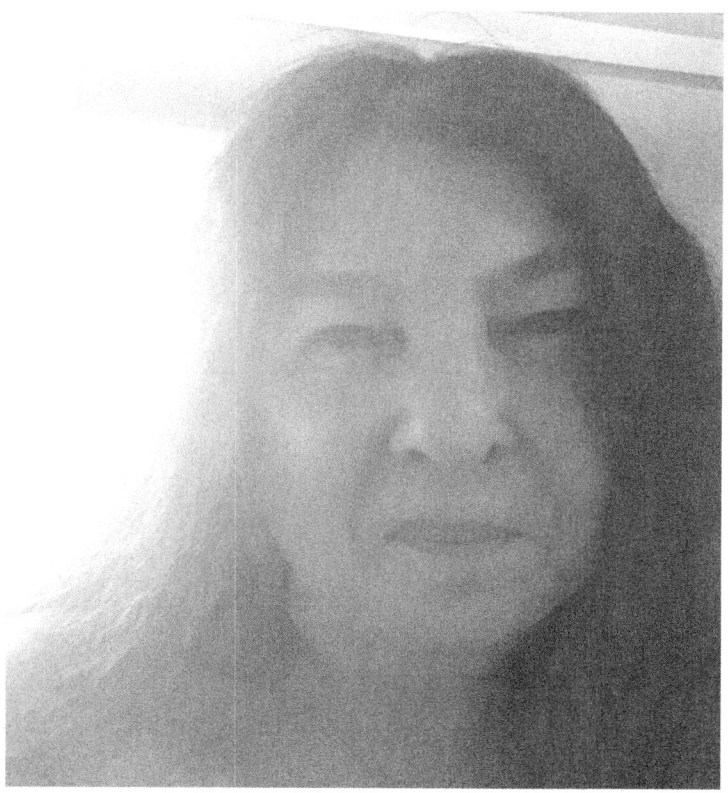

Author Lynne Noble at home

https://quintessentiallylynne.weebly.com/nutritional-medicine.html

Table of Contents

Preface	*Page 5*
What is cancer	*Page 10*
Cells of the immune system and some anti-cancer nutrients	*Page 32*
Melatonin, and vitamin D and their impact on NKC's and T lymphocytes	*Page 38*
Apigenin	*Page 57*
Quercetin, berberine and aspirin	*Page 61*
Fats in the diet	*Page 71*
Folate and pyroxidone	*Page 79*
Fasting	*Page 84*
Olive oil, Iodine and vitamin A	*Page 88*
Herbal Cyclooxygenase inhibitors	*Page 110*
Amino acids	*Page 112*

Preface

This book has been in the making for over a decade. It has gone through a number of changes in that time. I initially started off down the conventional route with well-ordered chapters on chemotherapy, radiotherapy and anything else that was conventional treatment at the time. I am surprised that I did. There are books galore on that same subject but none of those look at the natural healing power of your body if it is given the right nutrients to be able to effect that healing.

I was spurred on to bring this book to birth because of the increasing numbers of people who are reporting cancers at a time when medical help seems distant and uncaring.

I am sure that there are many who do care but in order to access that, one first needs a doctor's appointment and these, increasingly, are not forthcoming.

One individual who did eventually manage to get an appointment with their GP and was subsequently sent for tests which confirmed a diagnosis of inoperable bowel cancer, was actually informed of the results, over the phone when they were by themselves in the house.

Such an action saddened and angered me. What has happened to compassion and kindness at this time where life changing information has just been delivered?

Then again, people are often informed, 'there's no treatment available,' when really what should be stated is that there is no treatment available within what our particular organisation is able or willing to provide or fund.

There are so many alternative treatments with equally or greater efficacy. Equally, there are some very suspect ones where the primary motive is greed or prestige. People have some weird ideas but they are often delivered with great enthusiasm at a time of desperation for many vulnerable individuals.

Sometimes, it is right to let people go. The very aged are often ready to leave their time on earth and we should try and accept this. Others, until their diagnosis, were vibrant and involved human beings with lots to look forward to and lots to give to their families and communities.

In many cases, treatment will maim them, leave them with dysfunctional bowels and bladders, the removal of a breast, large scars and other evidence of human intervention.

Some people will willingly explore this route. Those women, unfortunate to have a familial form of breast cancer, elect to have their breasts removed.

Another lady, whose father had died of some form of cancer, had her womb and ovaries removed to lessen her chances of dying with cancer. I am not sure that I totally understand the reasoning behind that course of action but then I am not standing in their shoes.

People, unknowingly, develop cancers all the time in the same way that people develop infections. However, most cancers and infections are seen off by the immune system before we are aware of them. That's the power of a fully functioning immune system. You can never beat it for effectiveness provided that you look after it properly.

While we are keen to try coffee enemas as the solution to a cancer, most people will have never heard of Natural Killer Cells - those cells of the immune system which once activated seek out and destroy cancerous cells. Are we ever taught how to make and activate effective numbers?

All the immune fighters in the body which are composed of antibodies, white blood cells, T cells are composed of amino acids. Amino acids are needed to synthesise enzymes. Some have more importance than others. These include, glutamic acid, cysteine, arginine and glycine.

The use of free form amino acids is critical to the process of recovery as they are absorbed within seconds once they reach the gut.

However, there are vitamins, minerals and other natural substances which are crucial to the smooth running of the immune system too so we shall also look at these and what particular role they play.

As always, my main focus is on treating conditions through good nutrition although therapeutic treatment with supplements may be advised for a short period.

We shall start the book off by looking at what cancer is exactly.

Understanding the intruder enables understanding of how certain treatments may work.

What is cancer?

Cancer is accepted as a genetic disorder of somatic (bodily) cells. Genetic changes accumulate and this causes a change in the shape and form of a normal cell. This doesn't happen as a result of one change. A number of changes will occur over time building up to a level that will result in a cancer.

Different types of cancer will differ in the number of steps that are needed.

The abnormal cells don't respond to the regulatory signals that control growth and the programmed cell death that occurs at the end of its life. Programmed cell death is called apoptosis.

Other genetic changes may prevent genes from fulfilling their role. They may be genes that govern repair or suppress tumours. However, all cancers disrupt the normal function of the area in the body where it is growing. Cancers require nutrients for their growth and in parasitic style they take nutrients from the body often producing substances that break down (catabolise) the body tissues. This results in the rapid weight loss that people often associate cancer with.

However, when we refer to cancer it would be misleading to see it as one disease state with one underlying cause. There are many different types of cancer with their own set of characteristics and, as a result, require different forms of treatment. We know that people who smoke are more likely to get lung cancer and that meat eaters are more likely to be diagnosed with bowel cancer.

People oft cite how a relative – a heavy smoker – smoked for more than forty years of their life and died from something entirely unrelated to this disease. Perhaps there were other protective factors in play there that weren't fully understood at the time. Perhaps the smoker died from a smoking related disease but, in this case, it just happened not to be cancer.

What we do know is that cancer affects one in three people in the UK at some time in their life. The leading types of cancer in men are lung, prostate and colorectal cancers while in women breast cancer followed by lung cancer used to be the leading causes of deaths by cancer. However, cervical, endometrial and colorectal have now joined them.

As our diets change has the inclusion of different nutrients skewed the propensity to different conditions?

As more people go abroad for their holidays, this is reflected in the increase of melanomas – a type of skin cancer.

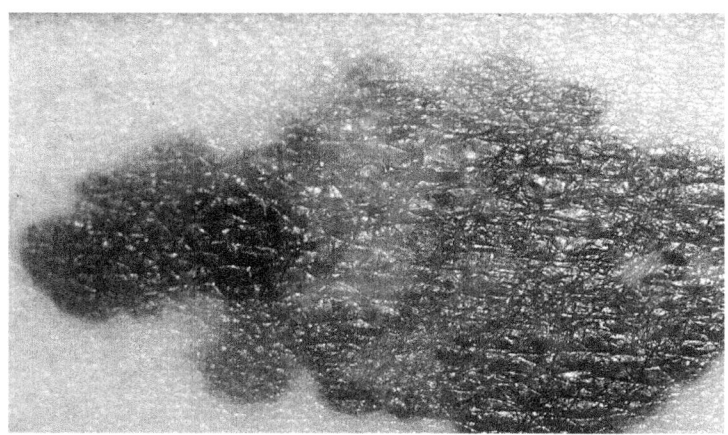

A melanoma –often attributed to damage caused by excessive sun exposure.

Nevertheless, recent statistics have shown that deaths from cancer have declined even though reported cases of cancer have risen. The latter, it is stated, is likely due to better diagnostic techniques and the larger numbers of people living to older age. Mention is never given to the fact that some cancers will disappear of their own accord just in the same way that we may develop a chest infection but in time the immune system will deal with it without outside help.

Cancer is confusing because cancer is not just one specific condition. There are over one hundred cancers.

Most are named after the tissues or organs where they begin. Lung cancer, for example, originates in the lungs and kidney cancer in the kidneys.

There are some cancers that begin in specific cells. Cells may be squamous (thin cuboidal in shape) or epithelial cells, for example.

Epithelial cells line the surfaces of the body and so are found on the organ surfaces, on the skin, lining the blood vessels and the respiratory and urinary tract, for example.

They perform an amazing range of functions including protecting, filtrating, secretion and excretion of substance, absorption and sensory roles.

Carcinoma's begin in epithelial cells.

Carcinomas that begin in different epithelial cell types have specific names like squamous cell carcinoma or basal cell carcinoma and each description helps us to understand a little more of what is going on and how it can be treated.

From this we begin to understand that cancer is not just one condition and following on from that, treatments offered by your consultant may differ widely from a treatment offered for an entirely different type of cancer.

However, the one thing that these cancer cells have is that they do not stop growing and dividing. That is, there is uncontrolled cell growth which eventually forms a tumour.

Normal cells control their growth and respond properly to external signals so that growth only ever occurs when it is needed.

At times these cells will undergo programmed cell death for reasons such as a response to irreparable damage.

They are also able to adhere to each other so that they don't migrate to other tissues. Cancer cells can and do metastasise because this 'brake' is not functioning properly.

Normal cells can also differentiate into specialised cells even when they arise from the same genome. This is not true of the cancerous cell.

Some cancer rates – such as stomach cancer – have decreased since the 1950's. Dietary factors may be involved but *Heliobacter pylori* has been implicated in the development of the disease.

Heliobacter pylori is a bacterium that can live in your digestive tract. If this infection is not treated, then it may lead to ulcers in the stomach or the upper part of the small intestine.

For a small percentage of those with this bacterium, stomach cancer will result.

Strangely, those who have lived in overcrowded housing conditions tend to be at risk from this type of cancer.

It may be that improvements in housing have impacted on the numbers of individuals who will eventually be diagnosed with this disease.

Perhaps it is the associated environmental factors that contribute to stomach cancer here. Is overcrowding associated with poverty? Poorer hygiene? A particular and less expensive diet any of which ingredients may potentially increase the risk of stomach cancer?

Are they more likely to smoke or drink to alleviate the stress of overcrowding?

Throughout the world there are differences in the types of cancer seen. When people migrate the pattern of cancer tends to change to that of the particular continent suggesting that environmental factors influence the type of cancer that is manifested.

As more countries become developed the pattern of aerodigestive cancers, seen in less developed countries - changes to that seen in the developed countries: that is, cancer of the endometrium, breast, colon, rectum and prostate become rifer.

Nevertheless, the occurrence of cancers worldwide is significantly greater in the developed countries than in the less developed.

Thus, the importance of environmental factors cannot be underestimated. Diet, of course, is a major environmental factor and we shall look at this in more detail. How does diet impact the genesis and development of certain cancers? What other environmental influences are there? This is what we should be asking ourselves? It is not just the domain of cancer specialists.

Perhaps we should take a look at some of the many cancers that there are.

> I suspect one cancer that most people have heard of is the melanoma.

> Melanocytes are specialised cells which give the skin its colour. I do not appear to have many. On a recent trip to the Amazonian rain forest, I was the only holiday maker who returned with skin as pale as they had begun their holiday with. I have red hair and an

'English rose' complexion, according to my grandmother. I have learned to stay out of the sun, apart from short and sensible periods, if I do not want to suffer blistering and peeling.

Although most melanomas form on the skin, other pigmented tissues such as the eye can also form them.

There is also a type of seborrheic keratosis which is often mistaken for a melanoma so initially the concept of ABCDE can be applied to assist in determining whether further investigation is warranted.

A= asymmetry – opposite sides of the blemish won't match in shape or size

B = border – is it ragged in appearance?

C – colour - a variety of colours such as different shades of brown or grey within the same blemish.

D = diameter – if it is larger than ¼ of an inch or is growing then further investigation is required.

E = evolving – that is moles that change in colour or shape, ooze, bleed, begin to scale, look red or inflamed.

Melanomas form only a small proportion of skin cancers but need to be dealt with quickly as they spread quickly to other parts of the body.

Leukaemia

The Leukaemias are cancers that start in the blood marrow which is where blood is made. Leukaemias do not form solid tumours but there is a significant increase in abnormal white blood cells which prevent normal blood cells from performing their job. As such, cells are not provided with sufficient oxygen, may not clot when required and there may be an increased risk of infection.

The four types of leukaemia may be categorised into acute or chronic or myeloid or lymphoblastic. The latter refers to the type of cell the cancer starts in.

Lymphoma

A lymphoma is a type of cancer that begins in T or B cells which are cells of the immune system which help fight infection.

Abnormal cells can be found in the lymphatic system.

Non-Hodgkin's lymphoma are cancers that start in B and T cells.

Hodgkin lymphoma refers to an abnormal set of cells known as Reed-Sternberg cells and usually formed from B cells.

Using light microscopy, they are huge compared to normal cells.

Brain and Spinal Cord Tumour

There are benign and cancerous (malignant) tumours. They are identified by the location where they began in the central nervous system and also the cells where they formed.

The above are the most commonly known tumours so we will now turn to some that are less well known.

Carcinomas

These are cancers that form in epithelial cells. Epithelial cells are the covering of the internal and external surfaces of your body. So, they form part of your skin but can also be found as part of the inner lining of your blood vessels, other organs and the bladder.

The most well-known of the carcinomas are the adenocarcinomas. They are found in the epithelial cells that produce fluid or mucus. Therefore, we can understand that breast cancers and colon cancers fall into the above category.

Squamous cell carcinoma – often referred to as epidermoid cancers - involve the flat squamous cell which are found just below the outer surface of the skin. They also line organs such as the kidneys.

There is also such a thing known as a transitional cell carcinoma. This forms in the transitional epithelium and are layered calls which can be found in the urinary system. For this reason, they are sometimes known as the 'urothelium cancers.'

Sarcoma

Sarcomas form in the bone and soft tissues of the body. These include blood vessels, lymph vessels, nerves, tendons and fat.

The most common cancer that is found in bone is described as osteosarcoma where the prefix 'osteon' refers to bone.

Many of the soft tissue carcinomas have long, convoluted and often unpronounceable names designed to indicate the location and soft tissue they are found in.

Multiple Myelomas

This is a type of cancer that starts in another immune cell – that of the plasma cell. These cells multiply in the bone marrow and, as they do so they form tumours in the bone.

This type of cancer may be referred to as a plasma cell myeloma.

There are many other types of tumour but the ones above are the ones that most people may have heard of, even if they know very little else about them.

Cancer occurs due to genetic changes which usually impact 3 types of gene.

- DNA repair genes

- Tumour suppressor genes

- Proto-oncogenes

If nothing else, this chapter shows that cancer is not one disease but consists of many. They will respond to different treatments.

There are a number of key immune system cells and nutrients which are cytotoxic to cancer cells.

Cytotoxic means that it is poisonous to cells.

Radiotherapy and chemotherapy are forms of cytotoxic therapy but - unlike nutrients - may damage normal cells in the process of destroying cancer cells.

The immune system can be divided into two parts.

The innate immune system

The adaptive immune system

Both play a part in dealing with cancer cells. As such there will be a brief introduction into these two complementary parts of the immune system.

The Innate and Adaptive Immune systems

The innate immune system is the first line of a General defence against invaders before they start an active infection. It provides a physical barrier to infective agents through:

Cellular – complement proteins attach to pathogens and mark them for destruction. They also make holes in the cell membranes of pathogens so that they are no longer viable.

Physical - physical barriers include skin, body hair, eyelashes, cilia in the respiratory tract, for example.

Cellular defences – consisting of secretions such as bile, gastric acid, saliva, tears, mucous and sweat.

Basically, the innate defense immune system's main job is to prevent the spread of pathogens throughout the body.

Often, if the innate immune system is healthy, it is enough to stop any pathogens from spreading in the body or the second part of the immune system having to spring into action.

The innate immune system is also required to initiate the more specific adaptive or acquired response which involves inflammation.

We will look at that later but it may be helpful to tabulate the immune system cells of the innate and acquired immune system so that they are easier to understand.

They have different roles to play in immune responses so some have greater importance when it comes to cancerous cells than others.

Cells normally patrol the body in a non-activated state. Once they are alerted to 'something that is not quite right' they become activated. The quality of activation is dependent on specific nutrients.

Strangely, a largely plant based diet is not particularly good in preventing cancer in spite of the fact that these diets are marketed as being 'good for you.' However, they do have some benefit as we shall see later.

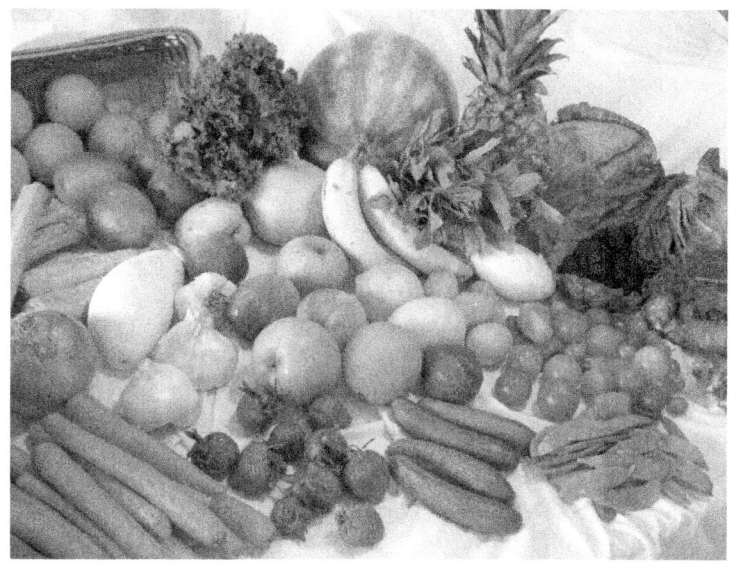

Many fruit and vegetables contain anti-nutrients which means that vital minerals are not generally bio available for the body to use. Trace minerals are important in tackling cancers

Table showing the characteristics of the innate and acquired immune system

	Line of Defence	Timeline	cells	Antigen needed	examples
Innate - non-specific	1st	Immediate response up to 4 days (96 hours)	Natural killer cells Macrophages Mast cells Dendritic cells Neutrophil Basophils eosinophils	no	Skin, hair Mucous Membranes Phagocytes granulocytes

Acquired or adaptive response	2nd	After 4 days/96 hours	T and B lymphocytes	yes	Inflammation Swelling Redness Pain pus

However, vitamin absorption is not inhibited.

We will discuss these in more detail later.

That is a potted history of the innate and acquired immune systems. They are your guardians. They need to be supplied with the correct nutrients so that they can protect you.

Now we will look at each individual immune system cell and its importance (or not) in dealing with cancerous cells. It is important to know who your allies are and how you can, through bespoke eating, enhance their ability to detect and destroy cancer cells.

[1]Cells of the Immune system

I am going to start with Natural Killer Cells (NKC) – aggressive 'don't mess with me' cells that detect and attack cancerous and pre-cancerous cells. They also deal with virally infected cells. Their importance in responding to cancerous cells is second to none.

They are part of the innate immune system.

Natural killer cells (NKC) can control many types of tumours and other disease causing micro-organisms. Natural killer cells have special 'pouches' called secretory lysosomes. They contain molecules which kill cancer cells.

They are able to secrete lysosomes quickly and kill rapidly if they have the right nutrients.

---

[1] Granzymes are enzymes produced by T lymphocytes and Natural Killer Cells which punch holes in errant cells, killing them in the process.

Diagram showing Natural Killer Cells in Non-activated and Activated form[2]

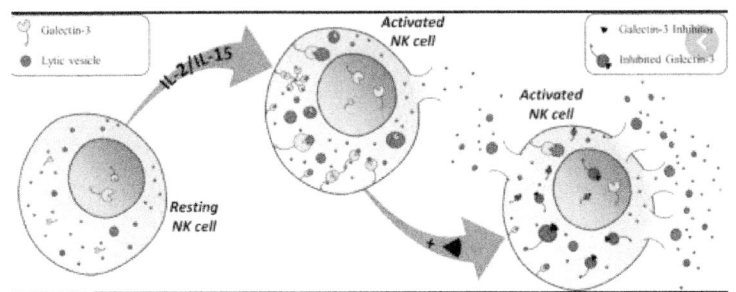

Nutrition really does make a difference to how many NKC's are made and whether those cells can be activated so that the secretory lysosomes can be poured on pathogenic cells.

The cytotoxicity of NKC's has been found to be significantly lower in a state of biotin deficiency.[3] The studies were conducted on those with inflammatory bowel disease but

---

[2] https://www.sciencedirect.com/science/article/abs/pii/S0165247817303607
[3] https://www.ncbi.nlm.nih.gov/pmc/articles/PMC6323526/

may have implications for those who are just biotin deficient and have other conditions.

Biotin is one of the vitamin B complex and is also known as vitamin B7.

More about biotin

Biotin is a water soluble member of the B complex. It was isolated from the liver in 1941.

It has a number of therapeutic uses including use in:

Seborrheic dermatitis

Treating skin complaints in general

Diseases of the scalp such as alopecia

Leiner's disease[4]

---

[4] Leiner's disease is a collection of symptoms (syndrome) which is characterised by seborrheic type erythroderma (on the scalp or diaper area) gastrointestinal disturbance and persistent or recurring candidal and staphylococcal infection.

It is, unlike many of the other B complex, quite stable so losses generally occur due to

Antibiotic use

Stress

Excessive intakes of raw egg white

No symptoms of excess intake have ever been reported. The Recommended Daily Intake is 300mcg. Biotin is also produced on a massive scale by healthy intestinal bacteria.

As a coenzyme it has a wide variety of actions which include:

Energy production and maintaining

Healthy sex glands

Healthy skin, hair, nerves, sweat glands

Deficiency symptoms are:

Persistent diarrhoea

Loss of reflexes

Muscle pain

Hair loss

Depression

Nausea and loss of appetite

Sleepiness

Smooth pale tongue.

Fortunately, biotin is found in a wide range of foods which include:

Dried brewer's yeast, pig's liver, vegetables, rice, meat, fish, organ meats in general, yeast extract, eggs wholegrains and wheat bran, wholemeal bread, wheat germ and corn.

It would be difficult to see how deficiency could occur unless due to poor absorption, chronically poor eating habits, prolonged stress or antibiotic use. I do not know of anyone with a habit that involves eating excessive amounts of raw egg white daily.

A vitamin B12 deficiency may also disrupt the effectiveness of the NKC's cytotoxicity. The cobalamins, of which B12 is one, are associated with immunomodulation and improved NKC cytotoxicity.

A Japanese study[5] of patients with anaemia and healthy controls found that vitamin B12 did improve NKC cytotoxicity. Further, research on rats found that when diets were deficient in vitamin B12, a significant decrease in the activity of NKC's occurred.

---

[5] https://www.ncbi.nlm.nih.gov/pmc/articles/PMC6323526/#B35

> In a nutshell, vitamin B12 appears to restore NKC activity and the normal CD4/CD8 ratio. [6]

CD4 and CD8 cells are immune system cells (T cells) of which the former has a 'helper' function and the latter has cytotoxic activity.

These lymphocytes of the immune system survey the body for abnormal cells and deal with them using 2 different sources.

> Induce death – mediated apoptosis[7] by forming pores in the cell through which granzymes and associated molecules can enter and induce cell death. Granzymes are enzymes produced exclusively by T lymphocytes and NKC's. They have a delightful habit of punching holes in tumour cells so they are no longer viable.
>
> The two pore forming protein family members are known as Bax and Bak (BB).

---

[6] https://www.ncbi.nlm.nih.gov/pmc/articles/PMC6323526/#B37
[7] Apoptosis is programmed cell death

Vitamin B12 deficiency becomes more problematical as you age. The stomach acid becomes less acidic but you need this acidity to separate the vitamin from its protein source so that it can be absorbed.

The lack of acid may well have something to do with a lack of thiamine (vitamin B1) as thiamine is needed to aid the gastric cells in releasing acid. Generally, a deficiency of one B vitamin suggests deficiencies in the other.

The absorption mechanism involves a specific protein in the stomach called the Intrinsic Factor and calcium.

Plant based diets do not contain vitamin B12 so vegans and vegetarians are at particular risk of deficiency. As this vitamin is confined to foods of animal origin then good sources are:

Liver and other organ meats (cooked lightly)

Fatty fish mainly but white contains some too.

Pork

Beef

Lamb

Eggs

Cheese

Vitamin B12 has further functions. It acts as two enzymes; 5-deoxyadenosylcobalamin and methylcobalamin. It is a nerve insulator and helps in the synthesis of the myelin sheath. It also detoxifies cyanide in tobacco smoke and some food. It is required for the synthesis of DNA where disruption is a risk factor for cancers.

Deficiency symptoms include a smooth, sore tongue, nerve degeneration (tremors, mental deterioration, apathy, poor cognitive function), psychosis, hand pigmentation found in people of colour, psychosis

Vitamin C as an enhancer of NKC's

It is understood that prolonged exposure to toxic chemicals may result in impaired NKC function. Many months after the exposure to toxicity, the NKC's may regain their normal levels. However, in some patients this is not always the case.

A study[8] was carried out which involved giving buffered vitamin C to patients who had been exposed to toxic waste.

After the initial blood sample was taken the 55 patients were give buffered vitamin C at a dosage of 60mg/Kg of body weight.

Blood was drawn again after 24 hours. It was found that vitamin C in these doses had enhanced NKC's by more than ten times in 78% of these patients.

It would have been interesting if there had been studies showing the impact of even

---

[8] https://pubmed.ncbi.nlm.nih.gov/9248859/#:~:text=Vitamin%20C%20in%20high%20oral,level%20after%20vitamin%20C%20usage.

higher doses of vitamin C on the activity of NKC's.

Research has found that patients can take up to many thousands of milligrams of vitamin C without reaching bowel tolerance.

Vitamin C is used up very quickly at times of infection and stress. Bowel tolerance occurs when the body's tissues are saturated with vitamin C. Once this occurs then explosive watery diarrhoea will occur. The dosage of vitamin C taken should be recorded and a 10% decrease is the recommended daily amount for your particular needs thereafter.

It's a rough guide only. Vitamin C needs will change on a daily basis depending on whether there are extra stressors, injuries and infections on any particular day. It is never an exact science.

Most people will reach bowel tolerance at around 2g (2000mg) but it has been found that patients with cancer have taken up to

60g daily and still not reached bowel tolerance.

Melatonin, vitamin D and their impact on NKC's and T cells

Melatonin is a hormone that the brain produces in response to lessening light. It helps regulate the body clock known as the circadian rhythm.

As daylight fades the production of melatonin increases and we feel sleepy. As light increases, the production of melatonin decreases and we wake up. .

Blue and white light impact mostly on our inability to produce melatonin which is why it is better not to look at screens late at night.

 However, any chink of light filtering through the window from a street light or from a clock will impact on the production of melatonin. Black out blinds are not a wasted expense when insomnia is a problem.

Getting enough sleep in a darkened room uninterrupted by blue light from phones or invasive street lights is important. Melatonin helps in the production and release of various cytokines in NKC's without which they will not be as effective.

However, the building blocks of melatonin synthesis need to be in place. Melatonin is made from serotonin whose precursor is tryptophan.

Tryptophan is an essential amino acid which means it must be obtained from diet. Some amino acids are 'non-essential' and can be built from other amino acids but tryptophan is not one of them.

The vitamin B6 (pyroxidone) is needed to adequately metabolise tryptophan. Further, given the fact that tryptophan is quite a large molecule – and is often displaced by smaller competing amino acids, a low protein diet favours its transport to the brain and kidneys.

There are, fortunately, many sources of tryptophan which include: oats, dried prunes, milk, bananas, fish, bread, lentils, peanuts, chocolate dark turkey meat and poultry in general.

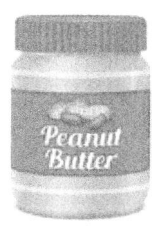

Peanut butter is a great source of tryptophan

As well as aiding sleep, these foods will help with the synthesis and release of vital cytokines which are poured onto tumour cells killing them in the process.

Cytokines are a broad group of small protein which are used to signal to other cells. They have a number of functions but for our purpose we must remember that they are used to modulate the immune system.

Activated NKC's secrete a diversity of cytokines. Some of them you may be familiar with such as

Interferon Gamma and Tumour Necrosis Factor.

Interferon Gamma is by far the most potent cytokine which is secreted by Natural Killer cells. It does not play a role in just antibacterial and antiviral activity but in anti-tumour activity too. That is, it activates anti-tumour immunity.

The cells surrounding the tumour are known as stromal cells. They are cells which are similar to connective tissue and they support tissue that encompass organ and other tissue.

It is these tumour stromal cells which secrete the functional cytokines in NKC's.

One of the functional cytokines is called interferon gamma. You may see it written as IFN-y. Other cells of the immune system such as:

Dendritic cells

Macrophages (big eaters)

Neutrophils

can also prompt the NKC's to produce interferon gamma.

As NKC's are part of the innate immune system, they respond at the very beginning of a well-orchestrated immune system response.

If there was some functional defect of the NKC's then there would be evident some form of immunodeficiency syndrome. This could result in the development of cancers.

In practice, these are rare. Most dysfunctional NKC's are down to poor nutrition which deprives them of, for example, the substances which act as activators or do not provide the necessary amino acids to make signalling proteins.

Communication is key between immune systems cells when they are coordinating a response to tumour cells.

We should now turn our attention to T cells which are a type of lymphocyte. They are able to kill cancerous cells although they are better known as the cells which kill cells infected by virus.

CAR T-cell therapy is a form of therapy that is utilised by taking the patient's own T cells which are then changed so that they will bind to cancerous cells and destroy them.

However, with sufficient vitamin D intake, this step would not be necessary.

T cells detect and destroy pathogens. However, in order to do this, they must be activated as they normally travel around in an inactive form.

In an inactive form they are a harmless cell. However, once they are activated they will seek out and kill anything they see as foreign.

The activator for the T cells is vitamin D.

Firstly, the T cells are exposed to the pathogenic material. Fragments of this pathogenic material is 'presented' to them by the macrophages.

Once the fragment has been identified as an invader, the T cells then attach to the fragment. The T cells then rapidly divide into many identical T cells. These identical cells are only concerned specifically with the pathogen that was identified in the first place. They would not recognise a different pathogen.

Chemical changes occur so that the T cells are sensitised to this invader and can deliver a bespoke immune response.

Whenever a T cell comes into contact with a foreign substance, it extends an antenna, also known as a 'signalling device.' It is not unlike a periscope on a submarine. This antenna is also known as a vitamin D receptor.

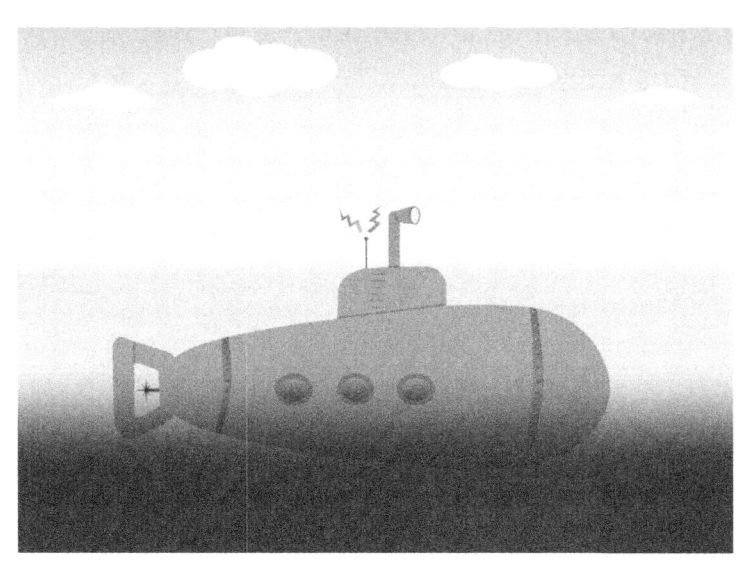

There are receptors throughout the body for vitamin D. Their ubiquitous nature shows the importance of vitamin D for whole body health.

All vitamins, minerals and other substances will have receptors but some of them are confined to specific bodily areas as they do not impact the whole body. For example, insulin receptors are found on muscle, fat and liver.

Now, this antenna/vitamin D receptor will look for vitamin D otherwise activation of the T cell cannot continue and immune system forces will not be mobilised.

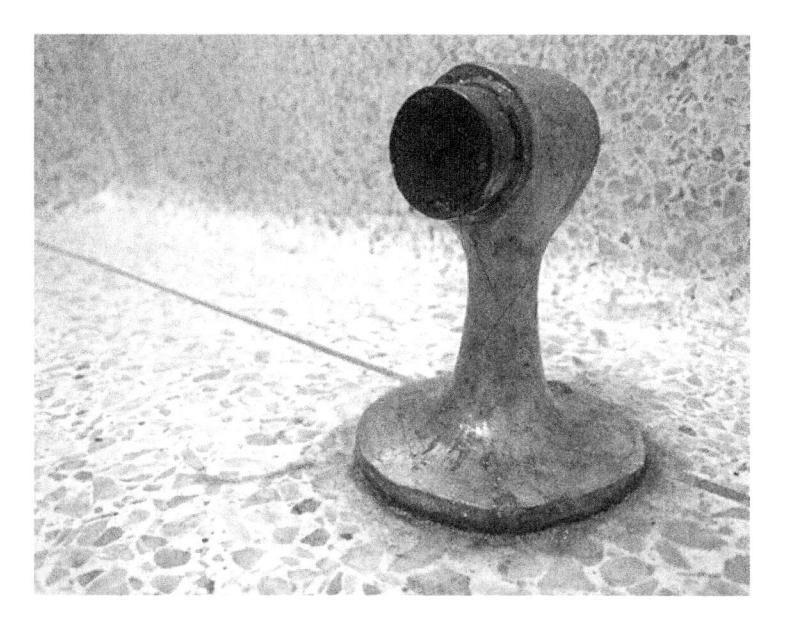

The T cell has an antenna, rather like a periscope. It looks for vitamin D. If there is not sufficient vitamin D, the T cell cannot be activated.

All T cells that are activated will then change into either:

a) Killer cells that will destroy anything foreign
b) Helper cells that help the immune system to acquire a memory so that if they come across it again, the immune system will recognise it sooner and see it off.

Unlike NKC's which form part of the innate immune system, T cells are part of the adaptive or acquired immune system. The adaptive/acquired immune system helps the immune system to recognise and deal with invaders.

Vitamin D is needed for the activation of both immune systems.

The rapidity with which active T cells can multiply is breath-taking but this can also have a downside if T cells fail to differentiate between host cell and foreign cells for a hypersensitivity reaction can occur.

Hypersensitivity reactions are found in autoimmune diseases. However, this would only occur in those with a genetic susceptibility.

Inactive T cells do not extend an antenna. Neither do they contain a specific molecule – PLC-gamma1 – which is required to deliver an antigen specific response for any particular foreign agent in the body.

PLC-gamma 1 is a protein found in humans. It is involved in the growth, the migration, apoptosis of the cell and proliferation. These are vital functions which are sometimes disrupted by mutations. If mutations do occur, then this increases the risk of cancer cell formation.

Many immunisation programmes work on training the immune system to function optimally but given the right nutrients, the exquisite choreography of the immune system works far better than any of the above could do.

Vitamin D has been found to be particularly beneficial for those with colorectal cancer and breast cancer. Other studies have shown benefits for those with small cell lung carcinoma as it decreases cell proliferation and induces apoptosis. Vitamin D is also known to inhibit metastatic growth.

Approximately 80% of the world population are deficient in this vitamin which is required for strong bones, regulating inflammation and activation of the immune system. It is one of the most difficult of vitamins to take in sufficient quantities through the diet.

Foods containing vitamin D are limited and what foods there are do not contain great amounts. As we get older we are less likely to absorb the nutrients from our diet. Vitamin D is no different so increasing age is a risk factor for a deficiency of vitamin D.

Most of our vitamin D is taken in through the action of the sun's rays on the skin but even this process becomes less efficient as we age.

Supplementation of 2000 IU's is recommended daily unless you have been out in the summer sun and had adequate exposure to the sun's rays and then you do not need to take it.

In the winter between the end of September and the beginning of April, 5000 IU's is beneficial. This should be taken in its active form D3 rather than the inactive form, D2.

The latter requires a number of steps to be converted to the active form. As age progresses, the conversion process is likely to be less effective.

Dietary sources of vitamin D are irradiated mushrooms, eggs and oily fish. However, supplementation of vitamin D should only be taken in conjunction with adequate vitamin K2 in older people who are less likely to make adequate amounts in their gut which is where the synthesis of vitamin K2 occurs.

Vitamin K2 is found in fermented foods including hard cheese and kefir.

Vitamin D is synthesised from the action of sunlight on cholesterol. Those on statins will, therefore, be unlikely to synthesise much vitamin D which may carry a susceptibility for some cancers.

When we come to the wonderful world of alternative health through bespoke nutrition, it would be remiss of me not to include apigenin – a little heard of but remarkably effective treatment for many cancers.

It is to this that I will now turn.

Apigenin

Apigenin is a flavonoid. Flavonoids are pigmented secondary metabolites. A metabolite is a substance which is formed when the body breaks down food, chemicals or drugs. When fat or muscle tissue is broken down the end product will be a metabolite.

The whole process of something being broken down is known as metabolism. The metabolites are then used as material which can be used for growth and maintenance as well as reproduction.

Apigenin has been found to be effective in many cancers and has wide effects upon them. These cancers include – but are not confined to –

Breast cancer

Liver cancer

Lung cancer

Melanoma

Osteosarcoma

Colorectal cancer

Apigenin is effective in inhibiting proliferation of cancer cells and triggers programmed cell death. It induces autophagy (self-eating). Further, it decreases motility of cancer cell and prevents migration of the cells. Finally, it prevents cell invasion.

There are a number of sources of apigenin. The beautiful herb chamomile is one such source.

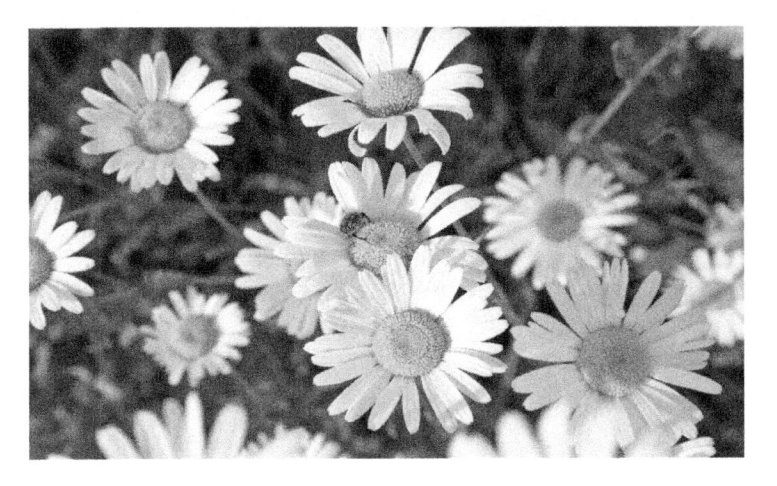

Found by the wayside and often treated as a weed, the beautiful chamomile is an effective cancer treatment.

Parsley, celery and oregano are also excellent food sources of agipenin with the dried forms containing much more of this active ingredient.

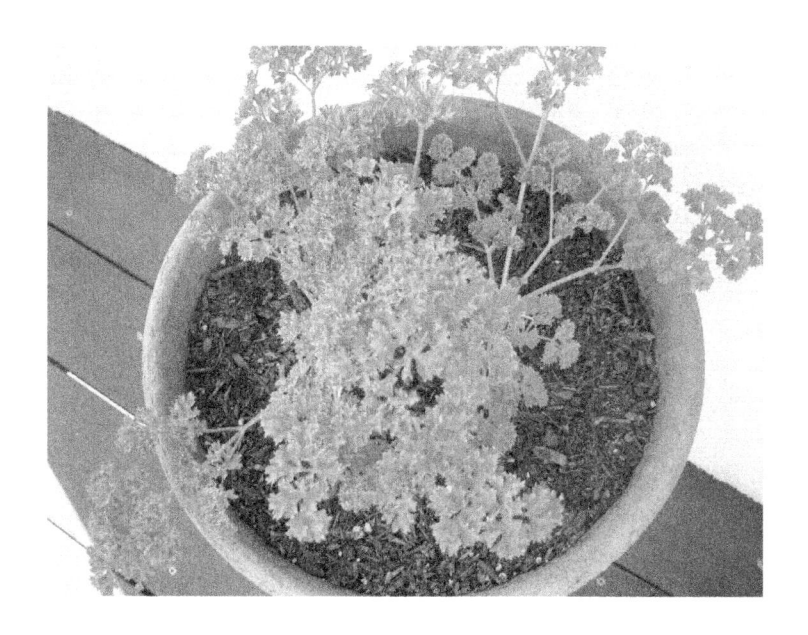

Parsley is an excellent source of apigenin.

250mg daily is the normal dose of apigenin to be taken daily for cancers. It is excellent in that it has lower endotoxicity than many other flavonoids.

Anticancer activity of APIGENIN

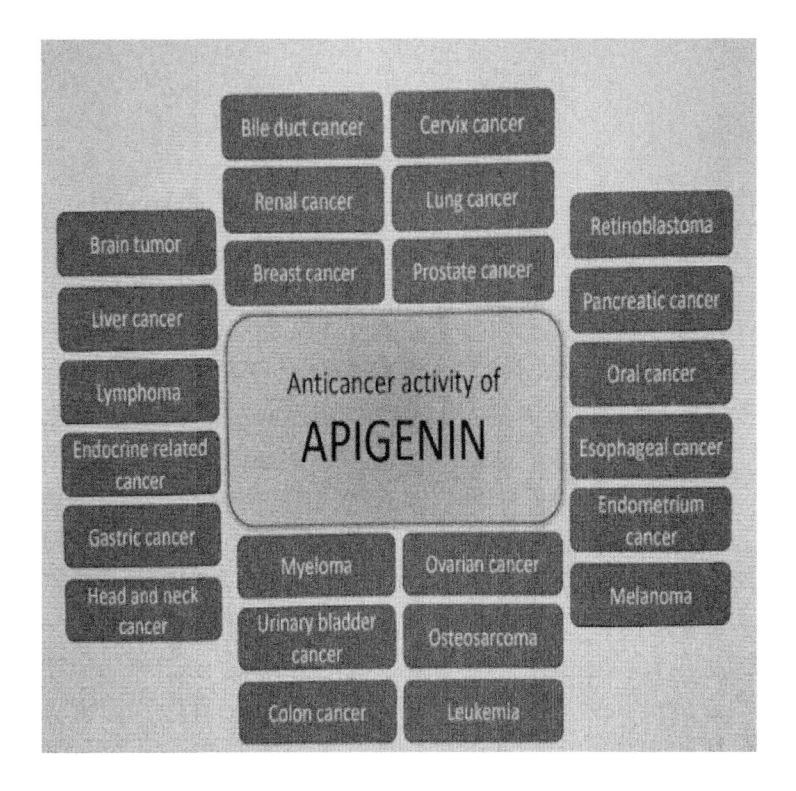

- Bile duct cancer
- Cervix cancer
- Renal cancer
- Lung cancer
- Brain tumor
- Retinoblastoma
- Breast cancer
- Prostate cancer
- Pancreatic cancer
- Liver cancer
- Oral cancer
- Lymphoma
- Esophageal cancer
- Endocrine related cancer
- Endometrium cancer
- Gastric cancer
- Myeloma
- Ovarian cancer
- Head and neck cancer
- Melanoma
- Urinary bladder cancer
- Osteosarcoma
- Colon cancer
- Leukemia

The flavonoids have excellent and varying properties and can address a diversity of conditions. Quercetin is a flavonoid which also has efficacy in cancers so we will turn to this subject now.

Quercetin has been shown to inhibit the proliferation of a wide range of cancers such as prostate, cervical, lung, breast, and colon.

Studies by Yang et al., 2005, Lee et al., 2006 found that quercetin inhibits cell proliferation by inducing apoptosis or by arresting the cell cycle.

A diet high in quercetin would include any vegetable belonging to the onion family such as leeks, shallots spring onions and garlic. Apples, wine and grapes are also excellent sources but there are many more too.

Supplementation of quercetin is generally taken at 500mg daily for a period of one month. A break of one month is then taken before resuming again at no more than 500mg of quercetin.

Mixing food sources of anti-cancer nutrients is always preferable as the combined effectiveness is greater than the sum of the inherent effectiveness within.

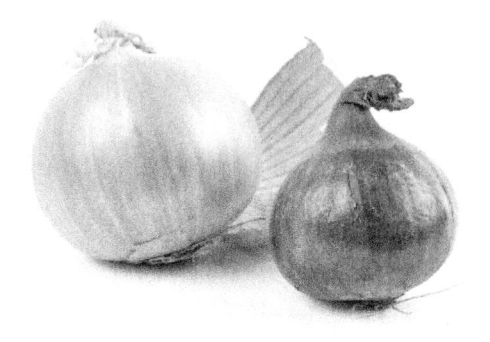

Onions are excellent sources of quercetin and can be included in soup, stews, pies, eaten raw in sandwiches.

Berberine

Berberine is a plant alkaloid which has been found to have clear 'inhibitory effects' on the following cancers.

Colorectal

Ovarian

Lung

Prostate

Liver

Like apigenin and quercetin berberine inhibits the progression of cancer cells and may induce apoptosis of the cancer cell.

It is found in plants like golden and those with bright yellow internal stems and roots such as you would find in barberry and goldenseal.

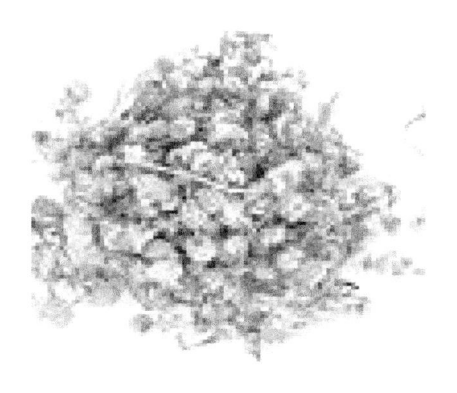

Dried goldenseal

Aspirin and salicylates

Aspirin has a long and fascinating history. The bark of the willow tree, which is where the active ingredient of aspirin – salicin - comes from has been used in traditional medicine for nearly 4,000 years. However, it was not until 1897 that aspirin was synthesised by Felix Hoffman, a Bayer Chemist.

The salicylates, precursors of aspirin, had been noted to have temperature lowering effects. These were described by the Reverend Stone in 1763, and consequently these observations were investigated and built upon.

The antipyretic effects of aspirin were added to when Pharmacologist John Vane found that aspirin also inhibited prostaglandin production confirming its anti-inflammatory action.

Later, aspirin's antiplatelet properties were discovered.

The story of this remarkable drug does not end there. More recent research has demonstrated that aspirin has a chemo protective action against many cancers including colorectal and breast cancers.

Dr Chan of Harvard undertook a study which suggested that long term use of aspirin for more than 6 years resulted in a 19% decrease for colorectal cancer and further a 15% risk reduction of any type of gastrointestinal cancer.

Aspirin demonstrates anti-tumour properties which include:

Impairing growth of precancerous cells

Inhibiting tumour cell division

Preventing metastasis

Preventing metastasis is extremely important as this is the main cause of cancer death. Aspirin prevents this action by inhibiting COX-1 thromboxane A_2 (Cox 1). Metastasis is prevented as Cox-1 blocks the adhesion between platelets and circulating tumour cells so that they do not attach to the endothelium.

More latterly, it appears that aspirin has an anti-oestrogenic effect.

Aspirin's amazing benefits for cancer sufferers continues to be investigated.

A major review of existing research undertaken by academics at Cardiff University found that those with a diversity of cancers who also took aspirin as part of their treatment could reduce death risk by 20%.

The review looked at 118 published observational studies of patients with 18 different types of cancer.

The results, when looked at in their entirety, included data from 250, 000 patients.

It was recommended as a supplementary treatment for those with cancer.

Aspirin may cause some stomach bleeds in some patients but compared to the risks of cancer, which is not adequately treated, the benefits appear to outweigh the risks.

Low dose aspirin was used at 81mg daily to both prevent cancers or the metastasis after cancer diagnosis.

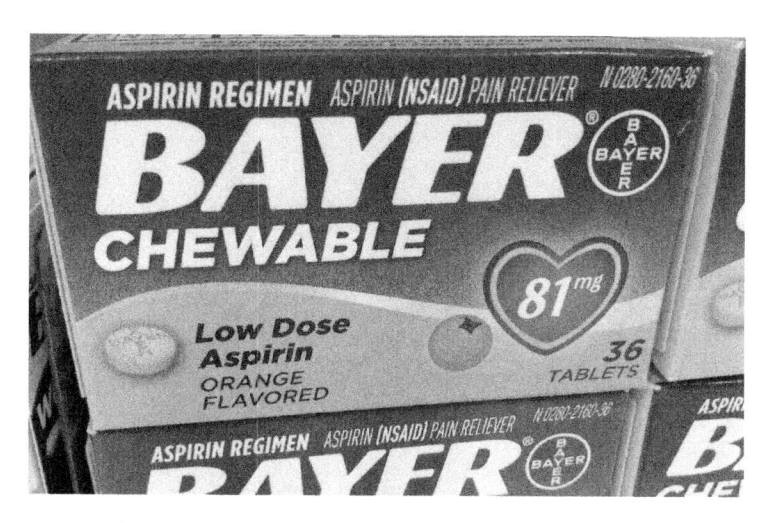

Aspirin has antipyretic, anti-inflammatory, anti-platelet, anti-oestrogenic and chemo protective effects

If salicylates are the precursor to aspirin, then including foods which contain these would have beneficial effects for cancer patients.

There is a huge list of foods containing salicylates – the major one is tomatoes. However, others include:

Mushrooms

Broccoli and cauliflower

Cucumber

Courgette

Spinach

Aubergine and peppers

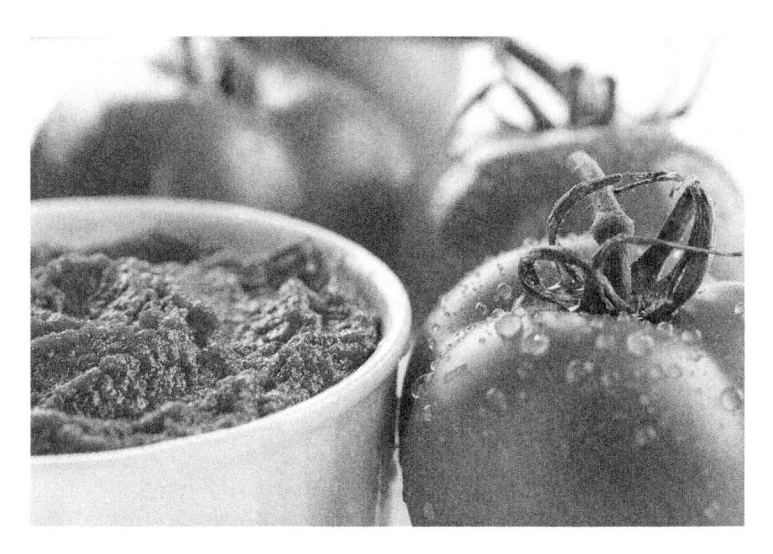

Tomatoes are high in salicylates and may be useful in preventing metastasis.

Some people find that they develop a sensitivity, or an intolerance, to salicylates. As such, they may not tolerate aspirin very well either.

The symptoms of salicylate intolerance are many and varied and include:

Headaches

Wheezing

Nasal congestion and runny nose

Hives, itching and skin rashes like eczema

Stomach discomfort

Swelling – angieoedema of the hands, feet and face

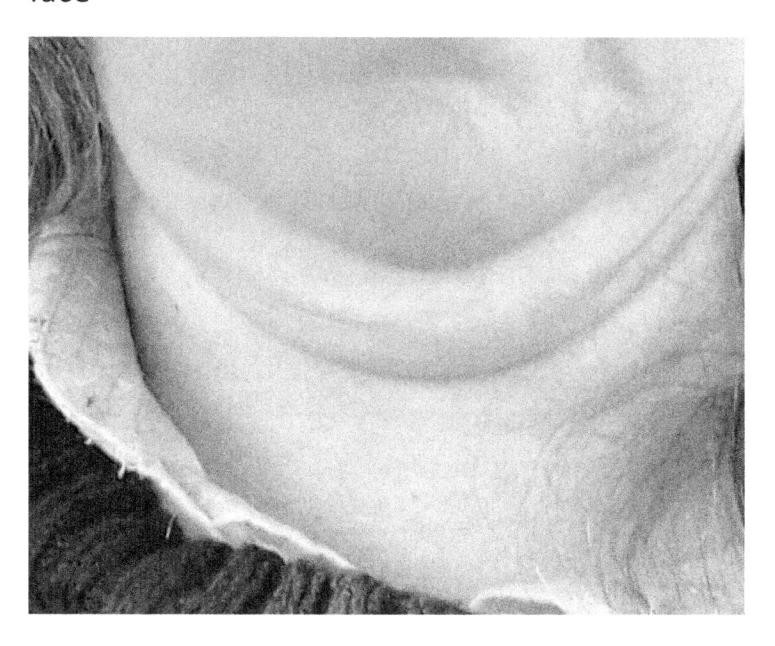

Angieoedema of the throat and face occurs with salicylate intolerance.

It is quite clear that nutritional factors are related to the cancers and this is borne out by *The National Academy of Sciences (Nutrition, Diet and Cancer 1982)* which found that 60% of women's cancers and 40% of men's cancers are associated with dietary factors.

Evidence does exist that precancerous changes may be reversible with supplementation. Calcium supplement may inhibit rapidly proliferating cancer cells in the colonic epithelium.

Vitamin C is known to reduce the levels of carcinogenic nitrosamines in the stomach.

Myths do abound about what may negatively impact cancer. For example, it has long been held that saturated fat contributes to the progression of many cancers. Does research actually bear this out?

Fats in the diet

A 1987 prospective study of breast cancer patients undertaken by *Willett WC et al. Dietary fat and the risk of breast cancer.* New Engl. J Med. 316:22-28, 1987) found that of the 601 patients diagnosed with breast cancer of almost 90,000 nurses who participated in the study, there was no positive association between:

Cholesterol

Saturated fat

Or linoleic acid

thus a reduction in saturated fat was unlikely to result in a reduction in the incidence of breast cancer.

A study[9] which had been undertaken a year previously in different groups of rats were force fed a mammary cancer inducer and either a high fat unrestricted diet, a low fat unrestricted

---

[9] Boisson-neault GA et al. J.Nat. Cancer Instit. 76:335-38. 1986

diet or a high fat restricted for 24 weeks found these results tabulated below.

Table showing the tumour incidence in groups of rats fed a mammary cancer inducer and either a high fat unrestricted diet, a low fat restricted diet or a high fat restricted diet.

Type of diet	Incidence of tumour after 24 weeks
High fat unrestricted diet	73%
A low fat unrestricted diet	43%
A high fat restricted diet	7%

The above results appear to show that the proportion of fat in the diet is not nearly as important as the energy intake of the participant.

This confirms previous findings that obesity and excessive calorie intake are linked to carcinogenesis while fat, as such, has not.

It appears that it is not saturated fat is the culprit in the development of cancers either. In Erickson KL, Thomas IK. The Role of Dietary Fat in Mammary Tumorigenesis, Food *Technology.* February, 1985 pp. 69-73 a study on rodents found that it was a diet high in polyunsaturates that were associated with carcinogen-induced mammary tumours.

This would make sense as saturated fat by virtue of its inability to react does not produce inflammation while the unsaturated vegetable oils are highly inflammatory.

If saturated fat intake is a risk factor for cancer, then we have to also understand that risk is not causation. It may be that as part of the diet overall, more calories as a whole are consumed.

When we look at takeaway meals nowadays they often contain a whole day's calorie intake and often include high amounts of carbohydrate as well as the inflammatory polyunsaturated oils.

In an observational study[10] of 50 colorectal patients and 50 healthy controls, it was found that the cancer patients were found to have an intake of 16% more calories than the controls. This was mainly in the form of carbohydrate which were fibre depleted sugars or fat with fibre depleted sugars. This ties in very well with the original mentioned study which showed that the high fat unrestricted diet (which contained unrestricted amounts of carbohydrates and protein) was vastly inferior when compared to the restricted high fat diet. (73% and 7% of tumour incidence, respectively).

---

[10] Bristol JB. Sugar, fat and the risk of colorectal cancer. British. Med. J. 291:1457, 1985

The calories in a gram of protein, carbohydrate and fat are thus:

Protein – 4 calories per gram

Carbohydrate – 4 calories per gram

Fat – 9 calories per gram

Looking at the above it would be easy to make the mistake that fat is the culprit in some incidence of cancer as it could contribute to excessive calorie intake but carbohydrate is the one macronutrient that raises blood sugar levels. When blood sugar levels rise, the body makes more insulin which helps the body store the extra calories as fat.

Saturated fat does not increase blood sugar levels nor insulin. Increased blood sugar levels and diabetes are associated with quite a number of cancers.

A consensus report[11] from 2010 found this:

---

[11] https://www.ncbi.nlm.nih.gov/pmc/articles/PMC2890380/

Diabetes (primarily type 2) is associated with increased risk for some cancers (liver, pancreas, endometrium, colon and rectum, breast, bladder). Diabetes is associated with reduced risk of prostate cancer. For some other cancer sites there appears to be no association or the evidence is inconclusive.

The association between diabetes and some cancers may partly be due to shared risk factors between the two diseases, such as aging, obesity, diet, and physical inactivity.

Possible mechanisms for a direct link between diabetes and cancer include hyperinsulinemia, hyperglycaemia, and inflammation.

Healthful diets, physical activity, and weight management reduce risk and improve outcomes of type 2 diabetes and some forms of cancer and should be promoted for all.

Patients with diabetes should be strongly encouraged by their health care professionals to undergo appropriate cancer screenings as recommended for all people in their age and sex.

The evidence for specific drugs affecting cancer risk is limited, and observed associations may have been confounded by indications for specific drugs, effects on other cancer risk factors such as body weight and hyperinsulinemia, and the complex progressive nature of hyperglycaemia and pharmacotherapy in type 2 diabetes.

Although still limited, early evidence suggests that metformin is associated with a lower risk of cancer and that exogenous insulin is associated with an increased cancer risk. Further research is needed to clarify these issues and evaluate if insulin glargine is more strongly associated with cancer risk compared with other insulins.

A high fibre diet may be useful in some respects. It may, for example, remove excess oestrogens and carcinogens. A 1984 study did show that cereal fibres were the only fibre that was associated with a lower risk of colon cancer. However, the problem with any cereal diet is that the anti-nutrients in cereals do inhibit vital trace minerals.

Nevertheless, even though the phytates in cereals bind essential trace minerals, they do not affect vitamin absorption and would also provide 'food' for beneficial gut bacteria. Further, they help balance blood sugar levels as complex carbohydrates help release sugars slowly into the bloodstream. As we have already learned, uncontrolled blood sugar levels are associated with many cancers.

Of course, the cereals contain good amounts of B vitamins and two of these – folate and vitamin B6 (pyroxidone) – have been found to have a positive impact on reducing mutagenesis and carcinoma of the cervix.

It is to these two vitamins that we will now turn.

Folate and Pyroxidone

An observational study found that 78 women who had had no treatment for cervical cancer, when compared to 240 healthy controls, had lower mean values of folate.

In a further double blind study, 47 women on combination type birth control pills with dysplasia were given either 10mg oral folate or a placebo. After 3 months, the only improvements noticed were in the group taking folate.

Moreover, another study showed that the cervical epithelial cells of women using steroid hormones and oral contraceptive agents showed megaloblastic features. Although there was no evidence for folate deficiency, the megaloblastic features disappeared with folate supplementation.

Smear tests, if positive, can form into one of two categories, either a megaloblastic smear or a non- megaloblastic smear.

The megaloblastic smear consists of segmented neutrophils while the non-megaloblastic does not.
The megablastic smear result occurs due to impaired DNA synthesis which will be due to a deficiency of folate and/or a deficiency of vitamin B12.

A deficiency of pyroxidone is also associated with cervical cancer. Pyroxidone is a co-enzyme in the biosynthesis of thymidine.

Thymidine metabolism plays a critical role in controlling the enzyme telomerase as well as telomere length.

As such, thymidine may have efficacy in patients who have potentially fatal degenerative diseases.

Where is thymidine found? It is found in
Fritillaria bulb extract.

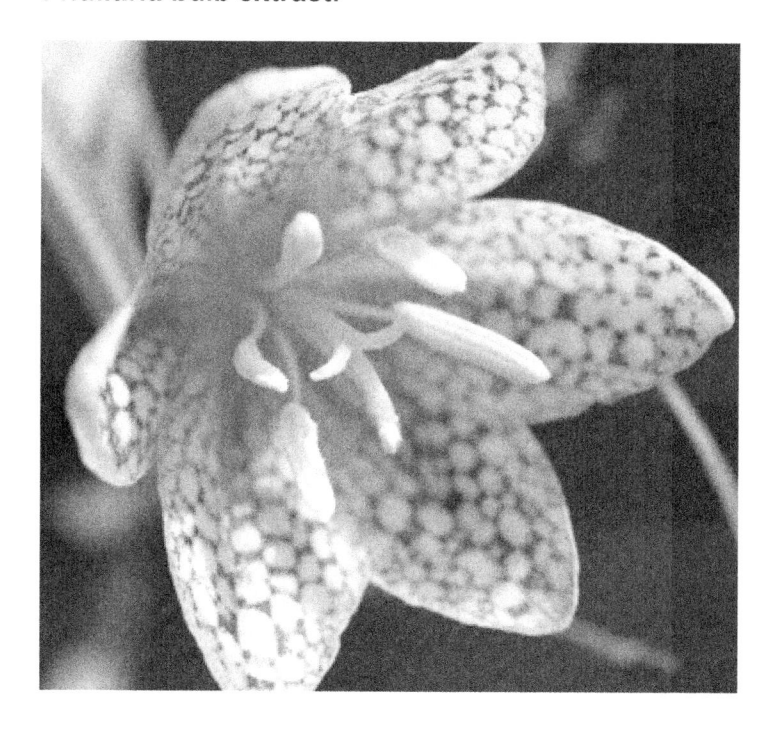

Fritillaria thunbergii – a plant that is used in Chinese medicine which contains thymidine, a substance known to extend life in those with degenerative disorders

Further, this beautiful and delicate looking plant acts on phlegm, removes toxicity, clears out abscesses and nodules and well as reducing heat in an inflamed area.

It is marketed as fritillary bulb extract although it is getting more difficult to source.

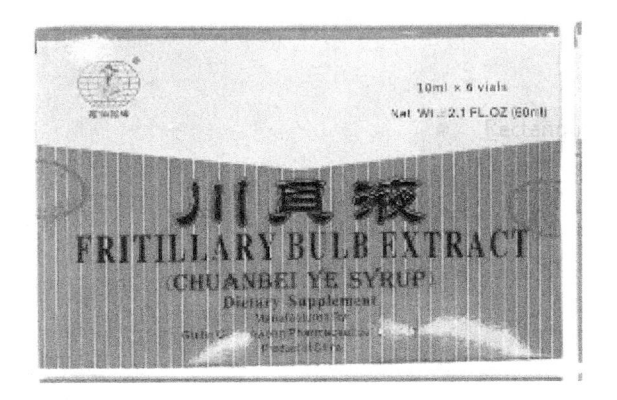

Fritillary bulb extract is a treatment for cervical cancer but needs pyroxidone as a co-factor.

Saussurea medusa is another medicinal plant which contains thymidine. It is also known as saw-wort or snow lotus.

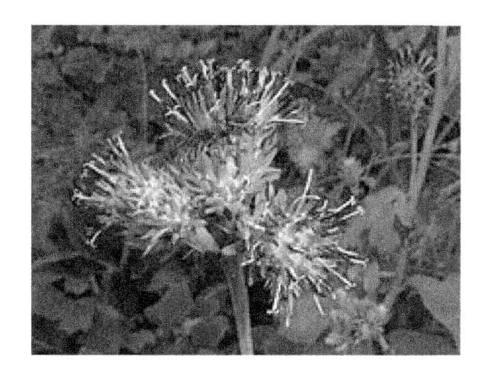

Snow lotus, source of thymidine

Now, we need to leave the subject of folate and pyroxidone and return to the subject of the role of excessive calories in cancer progression.

If, excess calories are linked with cancer progression, could it be that calorie reduction or fasting could impede cancer progress?

As it is, there is a huge amount of research on this subject and we will turn to this, now.

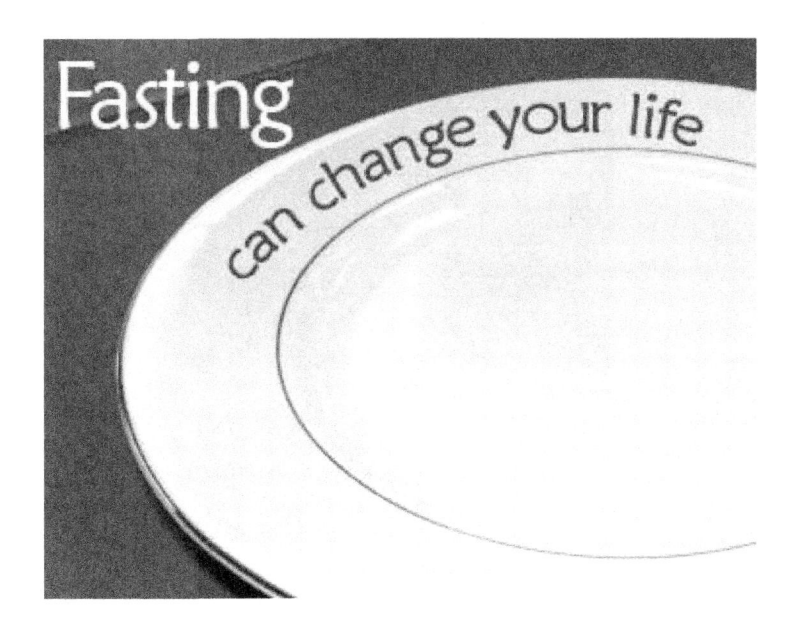

Fasting

According to recent research[12], it appears that fasting could play a vital role in cancer treatment. Fasting is able to create conditions that impede cancer cell's ability to survive and grow. Therefore, it is possible that fasting, as an adjunctive treatment, could increase the effectiveness of other alternative treatments.

---

[12] https://pubmed.ncbi.nlm.nih.gov/35848874/

The authors recommend this combination approach which apart from promoting survival will also help in reducing side effects.

During fasting a process known as autophagy occurs. A little understanding of this process goes a long way.

Autophagy

The value of autophagy as part of a treatment for disease conditions has been known for many years. Autophagy is a process in which old damaged cells are recycled in order to produce newer healthier ones.

Autophagy means 'self-eating.' In this process damaged cells are delivered to tiny organelles known as lysosomes. Here the larger dysfunctional macromolecules are broken up. This allows the cells to reuse the materials in the synthesis of new cells.

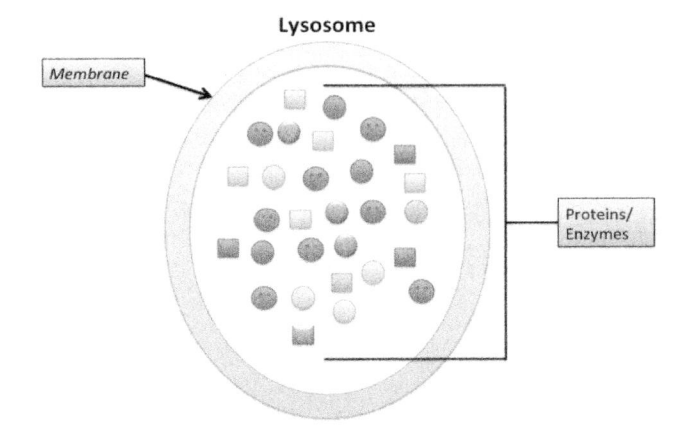

Simple diagram of a lysosome which degrades old worn out proteins using enzymes. They amino acids – building blocks of protein are recycled to make new proteins.

The removal of old and dysfunctional proteins is a necessary process in cellular repair, across all types, including that of cancer cells.

Intermittent fasting has also been found to affect gene expression which results in changes to gene function. These changes are related to longevity as well as protection against disease.

Further benefits are to be found in insulin levels. Insulin levels improve and insulin drops rapidly. This drop in insulin levels make body fat more accessible to be burnt for energy.

As we have already learned, research has shown that raised insulin levels increase the risk of cancers.

Fasting increases HGH-X5. This substance aids fat loss and muscle gain.

Given the many potential benefits of fasting, fasting for 14-16 hours twice weekly may be considered as an adjunctive treatment for those with cancers.

Why does autophagy work? Autophagy is able to inhibit tumorigenesis and cancer cell survival. It induces programmed cell death.

However, with regards to cancer, autophagy has another role and this is the opposite to the above. Autophagy is able to **promote** tumour development and its proliferation.

Based on this some drugs prescribed for cancer treatment have been made with autophagy regulation in mind.

You will know if autophagy is promoting cancer if you ask the consultant who is providing your care as this will inform the type of treatment that you are offered.

If you have decided to go down the alternative route and do not know your autophagy status, then this step should be avoided.

Olive oil, iodine and vitamin A

Olive oil should be avoided in those with breast cancer

You may have had to read this a couple of times believing that I have made a mistake but research shows that olive oil can stimulate malignant cell proliferation in vitro while essential fatty acids appear to have a protective effect.

An essential fatty acid (EFA) is one that either cannot be synthesised by the body or not in the required amounts for optimum health. They are therefore *essential* to the diet.

The two main EFA's that concern us are:

Alpha linoleic acid (omega 3 EFA)

Linolenic acid (omega 6 EFA)

These should be in balance but unfortunately there is a disproportionate leaning towards the omega (pro-inflammatory EFA's) in the human diet.

Studies[13] which found that polyunsaturated fatty acids may be tumorigenic are said to be most likely to be so due to their oleic content.

Another observational study [14] had similar findings.

---

[13] *Booyens J et al. Dietary fats and cancer.* **Med Hypotheses 17:351**-62, 1985

[14] *Wood CB et al. Increase of Oleic acid in erythrocytes associated with malignancies.* Brit, Med. J. *291:163, 1985*

The ratio of stearic acid to oleic acid in the Red Blood Cells (RBC's) was calculated for 60 cancer patients.

This reflects the desaturation or removal of stearic acid.

41 other patients with other conditions and 40 healthy participants were also included in the study.

The mean desaturation ratio for cancer patients was found to be 0.69

1.45 for patients with other diseases

And

1.5 for healthy participants

Further, the desaturation ratio was found to be significantly lower for the cancer patients with recurring tumours when compared to those without recurring tumours.

Another study[15] of epidemiological studies in women showed that oleic acid 'induces proliferation, invasion, MMP-9 secretion, activation of ERK1/2, FAK and Src and an increase of AP1-DNA binding activity in breast cancer cells.

What do all the above mean?

MMP-9 is a substance which has a vital role in tumorigenesis. It undertakes this by regulating migration and survival of cancer cell, promoting angiogenesis (tiny blood vessels which help to bring nutrients to the growing cancer cell) as well as aiding the formation of the tumour.

ERK1/2 is involved with growth and proliferation.

Src is involved in regulating many aspects of tumour formation, growth and proliferation, but is dysregulated by oleic acid.

A substance known as FFAR1 is also involved in cancer progression and oleic acid induces an increase of intracellular Ca^{2+} through the action

---

[15] https://ec.bioscientifica.com/view/journals/ec/8/3/EC-18-0543.xml

of FFAR1 in breast cancer cells known as MCF-7 but in MDA-MB-231 it promotes proliferation.

On the other hand, there are studies that have found that olive oil is beneficial to some cancers such as colon cancer but those with breast cancer should consider avoiding olive oil at this moment in time.

Other factors may also be at play when it comes to the development of breast cancer.

In an observational study of 5004 women it was found that those with a lower mean average of plasma vitamin E were more likely to develop breast cancer than control subjects. The patients and controls were matched by age, menopausal status, family history of breast cancer and parity.

Poor iodine intake is also negatively correlated with the risk of 3 cancers:

Endometrial

Breast

Ovarian

As vegan and vegetarian type diets are in vogue at the moment – and they are low in iodine – could it be that this form of eating is resulting in an increase in these cancers?

A review article on breast cancer found that women with low iodine levels are more likely to have symptoms of fibrocystic disease and precancerous lesions which have been rectified when additional iodine has been given.

Vitamin A is also known to inhibit certain cancers. High vitamin A intake is known to enhance macrophage functioning.

Vitamin A levels are consistently elevated in healthy centenarians[16] suggesting a protective role in immune system maintenance by retinoids.

However, retinol (another derivative of vitamin A with a different molecular structure to that of retinoids) which causes a slower turnover of skin cells than the retinoids, has been shown to suppress T lymphocyte function in vitro.

---

[16] https://pubmed.ncbi.nlm.nih.gov/10889454/

When activated, macrophages are an effective weapon against cancer. They can bring about phagocytosis (see diagram below). They are cytotoxic, that is, they can cause damage to cells.

So what are the sources of retinol and retinoids?

Retinol is found in animal sources such as meat, oily fish and dairy.

Retinoids which promote the M1 inflammatory macrophage are found in plant foods containing

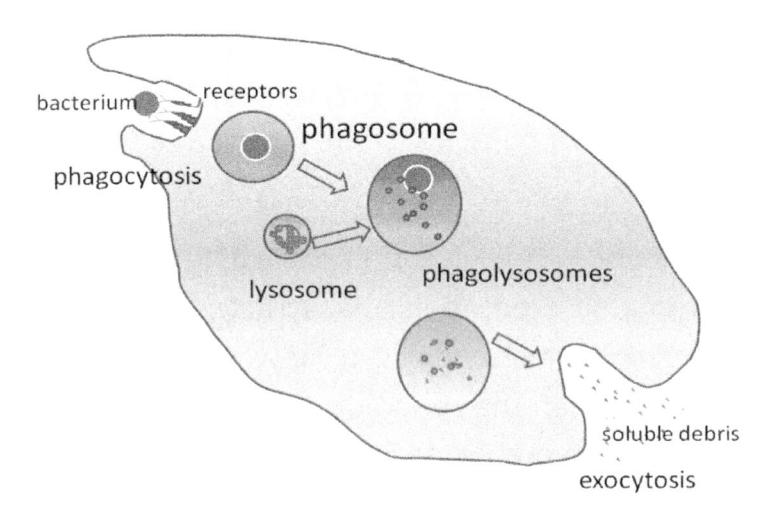

An example of phagocytosis. In this example, the macrophage is devouring a bacterium. It could easily be a cancer cell

beta carotene such as carrots, sweet potato, squash, pumpkins, cantaloupe, apricots, peaches and mangoes. In order for proper absorption they should be eaten with a little fat – hence the long established practice of adding a little butter to cooked vegetables.

Low serum retinol is associated with a diminished response to chemotherapy.

In addition, macrophages communicate with various components of both the innate and acquired (adaptive) immune system.

IFN-y is the most effective macrophage activating substance. It helps produce inflammatory M1 macrophages.

IFN-y is effected by activated T cells and Natural Killer cells. That is, infection and inflammatory substances get them ready for action.

Activators of the inflammatory M1 macrophages are:

Oleic acid (from olive oil)

Palmitoleic acid,

Polyunsaturated free fatty acids

Linoleic acid

Arachidonic acid

They are referred to as free fatty acids as the body cannot synthesise them and they must therefore be obtained from the diet.

Palmitoleic acid is found in palm oil but it can also be found in:

Meat

Dairy products

Cocoa butter

Olive oil

Breast milk (contains 20-30%)

Moreover, M1 macrophages are induced by bacterial components and NSAID's such as ibuprofen.

If vitamin A is able to inhibit the growth and proliferation of cancer – and we have looked at this with especial interest in relation to breast cancer – is it able to do this with other cancers?

A number of studies show that this is so. An observational study found that patients with cervical intraepithelial neoplasia had a significantly lower level of serum A. However, dietary intake was not found to be significantly different.

An observational study[17] of 374 males with cancer of the larynx plus 381 control those found to have a low intake of vitamin A had twice the risk of those whose intake was much larger.

Now, animal fats contain good amounts of vitamin A but our eating habits have changed

---

[17] *Graham S Et al. Dietary Factors in the epidemiology of cancer of the larynx.* Am. J. Epidemiol. 113(6): 675-80, 1981

and we have largely replaced saturated fats with the more (allegedly) 'healthy' olive oil.

Olive oil does not contain any vitamin A. it does however, contain vitamin E, excessive doses which are known to be a risk factor for haemorrhagic stroke and heart failure. In addition, vitamin E has not been found to inhibit any of the stages of cancer.

We can see how a simple dietary change can influence the range of health conditions which appear in society.

Some of the nutritional influences on cancers are better understood when tabulated. The table below is long but I hope, informative.

Table showing different types of cancer and their nutritional influences.

Cancer type	Nutritional influence	Any other notes
Breast cancer	diets high in poly unsaturated fats are a risk factor for cancer more than a high saturated fat diet 2) oleic acid in olive oil has mutagenic	

	properties. 3) high fibre diet protective. 4) high sugar diet is a risk factor 5)vitamin A is protective and enhances macrophage function 6) low retinol levels are associated with a diminished response to chemotherapy Vitamin E levels are found to be low in those with breast cancer Low iodine levels are a risk factor Selenium prevented or delayed the appearance of breast tumours in mice infected with a carcinogenic virus	

Intestinal cancer	Higher calorie intake in the form of carbohydrate is associated with intestinal cancer or a combination of fat and fibre – possibly as high fibre aids in excretion of excess oestrogen High sat fat diets appear directly associated with the incidence of colon cancer in blacks.	
Ovarian Cancer	Frequent fried food increases the risk Low iodine levels are a risk factor	
Prostate cancer	Smoking, lack of vitamin C Low serum levels of zinc are a significant risk factor Selenium levels are found to be low in this group	

	of patients	
Upper respiratory cancers	Associated with a lack of green and yellow vegetables Alcohol increases the risk	
Stomach cancer	Vegetable consumption decreased risk by 25% Alcohol increases the risk Smoked, pickled and cured food increase risk Low vitamin A levels are a risk for stomach cancer Vitamin C deficiency is low in all cancer groups but more so in those with gastric cancer	Vitamin C appears to lower mutagenic activity in the gastric juice. Another experimental study showed that 2g of vitamin C blocked nitrosamines in 10 students fed nitrate and proline. Results are consistent with the theory that stomach cancer is caused by endogenous nitrosamine formation from dietary precursors

		Vitamin C blocks the formation of nitrosamines from nitrite by successfully competing with amines for the nitrite.
Oesophageal cancer	Smoked, pickled and salt cured foods increase the risk.	
Cervical cancer	Plasma beta carotene is significantly lower, however retinol in animal products shows no effect suggesting some other protective mechanism is at work from plants. Low iodine levels are a risk factor Folic acid deficiency in cervical epithelial cells increases risk of cervical carcinoma.	

	Women on steroid hormones as oral contraceptive agents showed megaloblastic features even when there was no evidence of folate deficiency	
	A vitamin B6 deficiency can increase risk as it is a co-factor in the biosynthesis of thymidine, a deficiency of which can increase mutagenicity.	
	Low vitamin A levels are a risk factor	
	Vitamin C deficiency is a risk factor	
Lung Cancer	Squamous cell carcinoma linked	Vitamin E may enhance the

	to low levels of beta carotene	effect of cytotoxic drugs allowing a reduction in drug dosage.
	Levels of vitamin E have been found to be low in those with lung cancer	
Oral cancer	Deficiency of beta carotene increases the risk	Supplementation with 90mg of beta carotene for 10 weeks significantly decreased the incidence of exfoliated cells from the oral mucosa.
Laryngeal cancer	Low vitamin A levels are a significant risk	
	Vitamin C deficiency is a significant risk and supplementation has been found to increase the survival time of patients	
Large bowel cancer	Supplements of 10g of vitamin C	No chemotherapy.

	daily appeared to increase survival rate.	None of the patients taking vitamin C died during the 10-week study.
	Vitamin E supplements reduced stool mutagens by as much as 79%	Note, vitamin C should never be withdrawn suddenly as there can be a rebound effect
Neuroblastoma	Vitamin E inhibited the growth in mice and induced reversion of these cells towards normal	
Colon cancer	Calcium deficiency is a risk	Proton pump inhibitors and H2 antacids inhibit the absorption of calcium
	Vitamin D deficiency is a risk factor	People drinking soft water (lower in calcium than hard water) have significantly higher rates of colon cancer.
	Phytosterols in plants may protect against colon cancer	
Endometrial cancer	Low iodine is a risk factor	
Skin cancer	Patients were	

	found to have low selenium levels	
	Onions and garlic have been effective in decreasing the numbers of – and incidence of skin tumours	
	Lycopene found in tomatoes and red/orange vegetables and fruit has a protective effect against skin cancer.	
Brain cancer	Found to respond to curcumin	3mg per kg of body weight daily Higher doses can be given

Vitamin C 10g daily in divided doses when given to 'hopelessly ill' patients found that their mean survival time was 300 days longer.

Vitamin B12 and vitamin C inhibited the mitotic activity of transplanted murine tumours with a

100% survival rate. Microscopic examination of fluid from the mice showed some tumour cells in various stages of disintegration. These eventually disappeared. However, vitamin C and vitamin B12 given separately did not have this effect.

Magnesium deficiency is associated with risk of most cancers. It has been estimated that 300mg daily will prevent most cancers.

Selenium deficiency is associated with most cancers

Omega 3 fatty acids may inhibit the progress of some cancers. It contains EPA

Indomethacin - a cyclooxygenase inhibitor (COX-2 inhibitor) - has been found to inhibit carcinogenesis in animal models. EPA is also a cyclooxygenase inhibitor.

The role of COX-2 inhibitors in inhibiting cancers deserves a little more attention.

Herbal Cyclooxygenase Inhibitors

Apart from indomethacin as a cyclooxygenase there are many cyclooxygenase inhibitors. We have already come across salicin (in aspirin) which we learned had remarkable anti cancer properties.

Some of you may have heard of Vioxx (Rofecoxib) which was prescribed for arthritis and acute pain in general. It was eventually withdrawn based on data which showed that after 18 months there was an increased risk of heart attack and stroke.

Vioxx was effective but its withdrawal has left the way open for more natural cox-2 inhibitors.

Cox-2 is necessary for inflammatory processes which are needed to help heal damaged tissue. As we age, the inflammatory processes do not appear to dissipate as we would find when we are younger. They eventually become chronic inflammation nibbling away at healthy tissue and destroying it in the process.

Natural COX-2 inhibitors can help prevent this process and fortunately, for us, there are a number to choose - or combine - if you prefer.

These include:

Curcumin (the active ingredient in turmeric)

Ginger

Boswellia

Hops

Salicin (white willow bark and meadowsweet)

bromelain has an anti-inflammatory activity but, unlike the above, it does not act as a COX-2 inhibitor.

The curcuminoid content of turmeric inhibits something called 5-lipooxygenase (LOX) and cyclooxygenase which is the 'COX' already mentioned.

Curcuminoids are just as potent as cortisone for acute inflammation but while effective for chronic inflammation have greater efficacy in reducing acute inflammation. They are, for example, extremely useful for those having a flare up of rheumatoid arthritis.

Ginger exerts it anti-inflammatory and pain relieving effects via both the LOX and COX pathways. Its anti-nausea effect is useful for those going down the chemotherapy route.

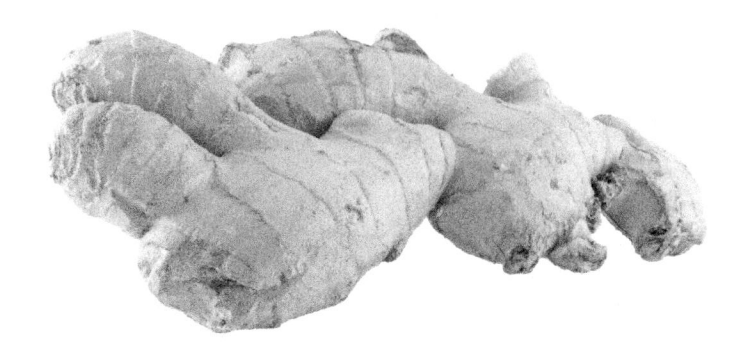

Ginger – A COX-2 inhibitor and potential adjunctive treatment for cancer

Boswellia inhibits the synthesis of leukotrienes. These are inflammatory compounds which are produced when oxygen and polyunsaturated fatty acids meet.

What we are learning is that there are safe and effective COX-2 inhibitors which have been demonstrated – via studies on Indomethacin – to inhibit the growth and metastasis of cancers.

We have now nearly finished our exploration of nutritional responses to cancer. However, we should not forget the amino acids. Amino acids are needed to build and repair, they are needed for enzyme synthesis, hormone production and life itself. When these are consumed by tumour cells then bodily functions cannot work optimally. This impacts physically and mentally.

We will now turn to this subject of amino acids.

Amino Acids

The immune system is dependent on amino acids for healthy functioning. After all, the cells of the immune system such as the antibodies, T cell, white blood cells, macrophages, among others are composed of strings of amino acids.

By the time that cancer has been diagnosed it is highly likely that the digestive enzymes will also have been affected so that there are not enough to break down food properly so that the patient can benefit from the nutrition in it.

Free form amino acids overcome this problem. They are absorbed in seconds by the gastrointestinal tract and while some may be snatched by the tumour cells, there will still be enough to strengthen the immune system as well as support enzyme production.

The result of this is that the body will be able to deal with the cancer via a greatly strengthened immune system.

A couple of individual amino acids are particularly useful in the fight against cancer. Arginine specifically is useful because it is a precursor to human growth hormone and, as a result, increases the size of the thymus.

Thyroid ——————————

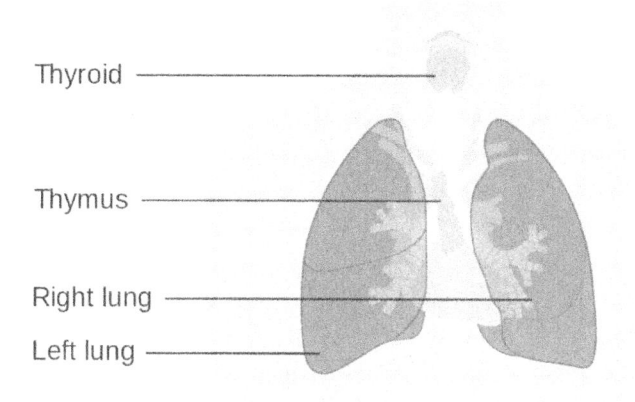

Thymus ——————

Right lung ——————
Left lung ——————

The thymus gland is important because it directs the immune system and response. Tests on mice have found that arginine supplementation inhibits cancer tumour growth.

The food sources of arginine are:

Meat
Fish
Nuts and seeds
Legumes
Whole grains
Dairy products

Glutathione is a tripeptide. That is, it is made up from three amino acids:

Glycine

Glutamic acid

cysteine

Glutathione is useful for fighting cancer as it works as a free radical scavenger helping to remove toxins that could cause - or worsen - existing cancers.

Cysteine always requires vitamins B6 and vitamin C for its activation.

The co-factors required for all 4 of the above for their optimum working are:

Vitamin A

Vitamin B complex

Vitamin C

Vitamin D

Calcium

Magnesium

Selenium

Table showing main sources of the amino acids, glycine, arginine, cysteine and glutamic acid

Glycine	Arginine	cysteine	Glutamic acid
Gelatin, bone broth, jelly, gelatinous cuts of meat (generally need long slow cooking)	Meat Fish Dairy Oats and wholemeal foods legumes	Ricotta. Cottage cheese. Yogurt. Pork. Sausage meat. Chicken. Turkey. Duck.	Generally high animal proteins: Meat Fish Eggs Milk eggs

These are, of course, not in free form so when appetite is poor then freeform supplementation is highly recommended as well as adding the above amino containing foods to the diet when appetite has improved.

Sadly, we eat very little glycine in our diet. It is the smallest amino acid there is but its impact is huge. The long slow cooking, the broths made from fish heads and chicken bones and tough cuts of meat, are becoming a thing of the past. Without glycine we cannot make the most powerful antioxidant that the human body knows.

Glycine also reduces pain, anxiety and enhances the quality of sleep.

Nature has provided an abundance of healing foods and herbs. They are all around us be we have long forgotten their healing properties and need to become acquainted with them again.

They are gentle in action but strong in effect. Whatever treatment route the cancer patient takes there should be a number of avenues that are available to be considered before making a decision.

This book is intended to provide one of those routes.

Additional chapter

> Vitamin K2 and its inverse association with many cancers

Many people may not be aware of the inverse association of vitamin K2 and the manifestation of many cancers. Vitamin K2   consists of a group of 9 forms which are known as menaquinones. They are synthesised from gut bacteria - also known as intestinal microbiota - apart from MK-4 which is converted from vitamin K1 –phylloquinone.

 Vitamin K2 is, of course, found in fermented foods such as yogurt, natto, goose liver pate and cheese. Indeed, the consumption of cheese has been found to be the protecting factor for many cancers as a fermented food which helps the increase of the synthesis of vitamin K2. Studies have also shown that there is an inverse association with advanced prostate cancer. It appears that the more   full fat dairy that is consumed the less likely you are to suffer from advanced prostate cancer.

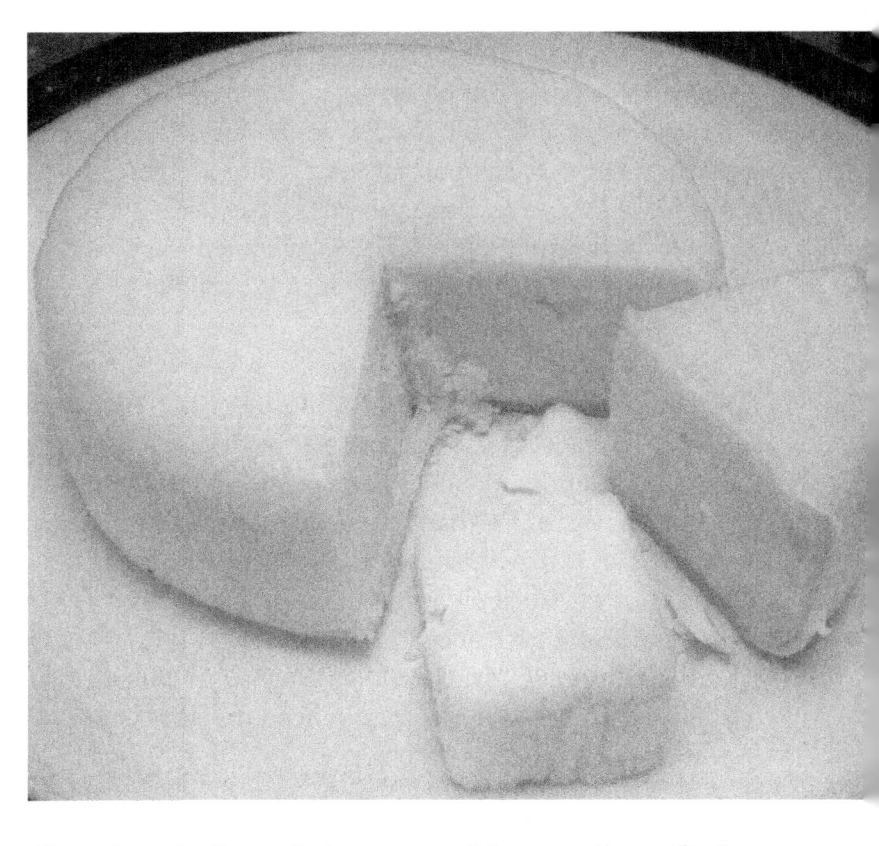

Cheese is protective against cancers as it increases the synthesis of vitamin K2

However, vitamin K2 is not just protective against prostate cancer. The protective effects also extend to ovarian, liver, lung, nose, throat and mouth cancers as well as stomach, colon, breast and bowel. Quite an impressive list of protection against cancers for vitamin K2.

The European Prospective Investigation into Cancer and Nutrition (EPIC) undertook a study which involved 24,000 patients over a period of 10 years. They found that those with the highest intake of K2 were associated with a significantly reduced risk of developing cancer with the overall death from cancer being 30% lower. Thus a diet high in vitamin K2 significantly helps prevent cancer.

Liver cancer

Vitamin K2 also prevents cancer in women with hepatitis and helps induce the death of liver tumour cells which suggests that vitamin K2 is important in inhibiting tumour growth and invasiveness.

Additionally, during clinical trials for the effectiveness of using vitamin K2 for cirrhosis the results were so positive that it is recommended that all patients with hepatitis take a K2 supplement.

Lymph Cancers

In a paper entitled **Vitamin K may cut lymph cancer risk: Us study**

21-April-2010 By Stephen Daniells

Increased intakes of vitamin K from dietary and supplementary sources may reduce the risk of cancers of the lymphatic system according to new findings from the Mayo clinic.[18]

Non-Hodgkin lymphoma (NHL) is a common cancer which occurs in about 4% of the population with a cancer in the United States. Males tend to account for the greater percentage of Non-Hodgkin Lymphoma with estimates of nearly 45,000 males diagnosed to approximately 36,000 females for 2023 figures.

Approximately 75% of those with NHL will have survived at 5 years but, of course, treatments and loss of time spent doing things you want to do, impact greatly those 5 years.

Chemotherapy does not come without some distressing side effects although some patients appear to suffer no side effects whatsoever. When vitamin K2 is able to reduce the risk of many cancers, including lymphomas, it makes sense to eat a wide variety of fermented food on a daily basis especially if there appears to be a familial predisposition to cancers. Moreover, those who were diagnosed with cancer were less likely to die

---

[18] https://www.nutraingredients.com/Article/2010/04/21/Vitamin-K-may-cut-lymph-cancer-risk-US-study

from it and this was inversely connected to the amount of vitamin K2 in the diet.

Leukaemia

Many studies have been undertaken on the impact of vitamin K2 on leukaemia which is cancer of blood and bone marrow and in which there is a pathological increase in white blood cells. Leukaemia is the main cancer found in children and causes death in about 50% of those who have it.

The findings in research - with regards to vitamin K2 and its treatment of leukaemia - are very encouraging and support high dose vitamin K2 in the treatment of leukaemia and subsequently, full remission. Menaquinone induced apoptosis in all leukaemia cells. Apoptosis is a term used for cell death and appears to have similar effects whether the cancer cells are cultured in the laboratory or found in blood samples.

Menaquinone also encourages rogue leukaemia cells to differentiate to harmless white blood cells.

Now, menaquinone is generally measured in micrograms (mcg) where 1000mcg are required to make one milligram (mg). Although a recommended daily intake has not been established for vitamin K, it is thought that between 90-120 mcg is about the right amount to prevent bleeding. As usual a recommended daily amount is based on one of the many functions of vitamin K which may require far lower amounts than is required for other functions in the body.

Whenever you come across a recommended daily intake, research why it was set at that amount. It was generally set as the minimum amount needed to avoid a **specific** deficiency symptom without any reference to the **other functions** that a specific nutrient may be involved in and which require much higher intakes. For example, vitamin K2 is required for the health of

The skin

Bone metabolism

Brain function

Prevention of blood vessel calcification

But much lower intake of vitamin K2 may be needed for healthy skin as opposed to bone metabolism. This may explain why, when a deficiency of any nutrient occurs, only some symptoms are manifested. Nevertheless, genetics also dictate which symptoms may be apparent.

A particular case of interest was that of a 72-year-old woman who was diagnosed with acute leukaemia. Although standard treatment did result in a remission, a relapse followed 8 months later. In addition to her normal treatment, 20mg of menaquinone was added daily to her regime. After 2 months a complete remission occurred.

Menaquinone works well with the fat soluble vitamins A and D with vitamin K2 and vitamin D working together to prevent cytopenia – a side effect of chemotherapy where the infection fighting cells are much reduced. It needs to be repeated that vitamin K is also a fat soluble vitamin and requires fat for its absorption as do vitamin A and D.

Although menaquinone in the form of MK-4 has poor bioavailability, it is the form of vitamin K2 which was given to patients as opposed to the more bio available form found in MK-7. Why this was so? I do not have any idea. Nevertheless, it was the form that specifically addressed leukaemia and many other common cancers effectively.

No Tolerable Upper Limit has been found for vitamin K – no toxicity whatsoever whatever the form of vitamin K either from food or supplements.

Dietary deficiencies of vitamin K2 may occur due to problems with the gut since menaquinones (apart from MK-4) are generally synthesised by bacteria. Problems with the gut may include surgery or prolonged antibiotic use. However, fermented foods and animal based foods do provide some.

MK-4 specifically differs in that it is produced endogenously from phylloquinone (vitamin K1) and this process does not involve any bacterial action whatsoever. Phylloquinone is found in vegetables – mainly leafy greens – and some fruit.

Dietary fats and fat soluble vitamins (vitamins ADEK) are incorporated into micelles. Micelles are very tiny particles and are soluble in water. They can curl up into a ball shape and within this they are able to carry substances to where they are needed in the body.

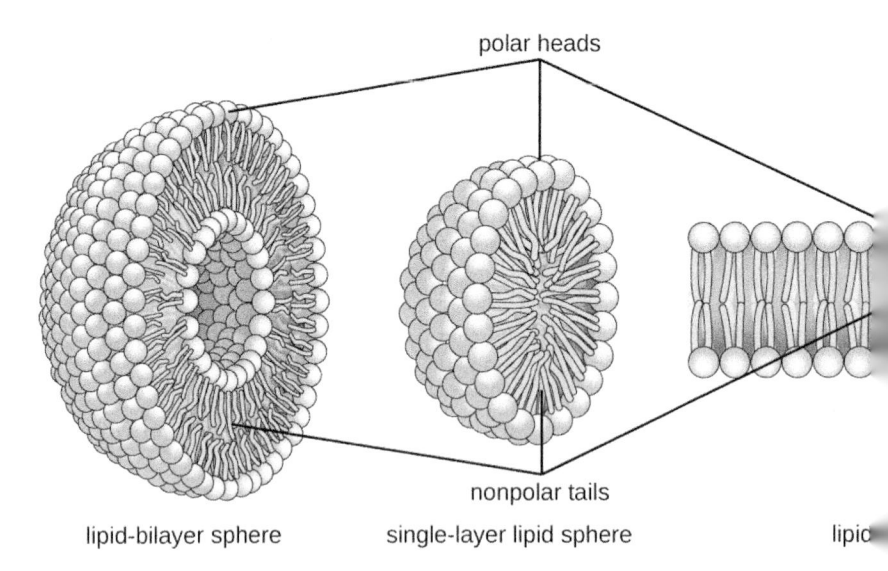

polar heads

nonpolar tails

lipid-bilayer sphere   single-layer lipid sphere   lipid

Micelles curled up and flat.

Vitamin K is also transported in micelles to where it is needed. However, it is also dependent on bile and pancreatic enzymes as part of this process, before it is absorbed by intestinal cells known as enterocytes. Its journey is still not finished because it is then integrated into chylomicrons which are much larger particles made by the intestine. Their function is to carry triglycerides and cholesterol to the liver and tissues.

When vitamin K is transported to the liver it is parcelled into a very low density lipoproteins (VLDL) and it is in this form that it is circulated around the body. Statins not only lower LDL but VLDL as well. It does this by hastening the clearance of lipoproteins as well as reducing the production and release of them in the liver.

You may want to question whether this is a good thing considering that high levels of vitamin K are associated with lower risks of cancer and an increased survival rate if cancer does manifest itself.

Colorectal Cancer

The benefits of vitamin K2 has been known for well over a decade. For example, a study [19] from 2007 makes

---

[19] https://pubmed.ncbi.nlm.nih.gov/17611688/

reference to that fact that a number of studies have shown that vitamin K holds antitumor properties on cells showing abnormal and uncontrolled growth (these are commonly referred to as neoplastic cell lines)

In this particular study, examination of the effect of vitamin K on colorectal cancer took place both in vivo and in vitro. It was noted that vitamin K2 (along with K3 and K5) inhibited the proliferation of colon 26 cells. The colon 26 cells are a particular cell line that was originally isolated from the large intestine of a mouse. It is frequently used in cancer research. The suppression of the C26 cells occurred in a dose dependent manner. Therefore, the more vitamin K2 that was available the more that programmed cell death occurred.

Ovarian cancer

There is generally delayed diagnosis with ovarian cancer since the symptoms overlap with so many other conditions so it is good news that vitamin K2 is able to depolarise mitochondrial membranes through production of hydrogen peroxide which induces apoptosis of the rogue cancer cells.

Cell depolarisation also known as membrane depolarisation occurs when there is a shift in electrical charge so the cell is less negatively charged when compared to its environment

Hydrogen peroxide is an oxidising agent and causes cell damage and eventually cell death so K2's help in this process is invaluable for combatting cancers including ovarian cancer.

Pancreatic cancer

While many studies have found that it is the menaquinone MK-4 that comes under the umbrella of vitamin K2, it has been found that a dietary intake of vitamin K1 is inversely associated with the risk of pancreatic cancer. This begs the question of why vitamin K is not prescribed as a potential treatment as it has extremely low toxicity and great efficacy?

The quinone part of vitamin K is used in many cancer drugs. The synthetic K3 appears to have significant efficacy as well but it is mainly K2 which induces apoptosis in cancer cells. K2 also induces autophagy or self-eating of the cancer cell. There are numerous studies which show that K2 works well synergistically with other compounds which have anti cancer activity. It however, has an antagonistic effect when used in conjunction with methotrexate.

Vitamin C also works synergistically with vitamin K3. When paired there is a massive increase in oxidative stress alongside a lowering of the membrane potential of the mitochondria (little organelles which are the powerhouses of cells). This triggers the death of tumour cells.

In order to obtain maximum benefit from the various forms of vitamin K, here is a reminder.

Dietary vitamin K1 is inversely associated with the risk of pancreatic cancer.

Vitamin K2 is able to induce cell death in many types of cancer but also has the ability to induce differentiation from cancer cell to harmless non-cancerous cell. Vitamin K1 and the MK-4 are obtained from a diet rich in fruit and vegetables (remember that MK-4 is not of bacterial origin although the other menaquinones are and is made from phylloquinone)

There is a synthetic form of vitamin K known as menadione which is a precursor of MK-4. Such a supplement has some toxic effects and is only used in animal feed and pet food.

Sources of phylloquinone

It is important to know the sources of phylloquinone since MK-4 is the end product of a conversion process of phylloquinone to the menaquinone MK-4.

The main sources are:

Vegetables especially green leafy vegetable and some fruits. If markedly increasing green leafy vegetables, then you need to be aware that they also contain goitregens.

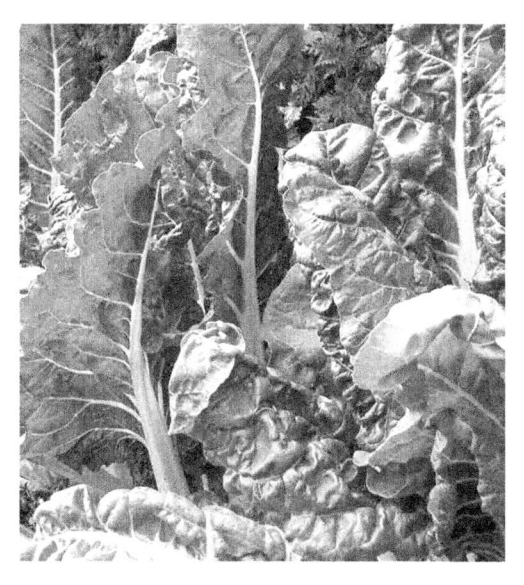

Green leafy vegetables contain phylloquinone which is converted to MK-4. However, they also contain goitregens and may not be suitable for those with a thyroid disorder if taken if large quantities

Goitregens are also known as anti-nutrients and, for people with thyroid dysfunction, a high intake may prevent iodine from being able to enter the thyroid. Iodine is needed to synthesise thyroid hormones so for people with a susceptibility to thyroid dysfunction, they need to be aware that increasing foods contain goitregens may alter their thyroxine levels. This, of course, can be treated, but for people with a susceptibility to problematical thyroxine synthesis, supplements may be useful.

Animal proteins like meat, eggs and dairy tend to have useful amounts of menaquinone but low amounts of phylloquinone.

Final comment on this subject

In all of the hundreds of stories that I have listened to from people diagnosed with cancer, not one has ever been advised to change their diet – not one who has been advised to increase their intake of green leafy veg and fruit and vegetable in general. Not one has been advised about the benefits of vitamin K2 or that its origins lay in its conversion of phylloquinone to MK-4. Why not? I have to ask this because when you have a treatment that comes with any negative side effects, is non-toxic, is easily available and cheap, then it does not make sense to withhold this information from the patient. Yet it is not imparted and may be deliberately withheld. After all vitamin K2 is easy to source and cheap, there is little, if any, profit to be made from it when the fields are full of green leafy plants just ready to be picked.

We seem to have come a long way from the times when it was quite normal to pick a basket full of green leafy nettles to make nettle and potato soup. Decades ago people knew the value of nettles. I recall making nettle and potato soup for my children with some wild garlic and some stock from some chicken bones that I had boiled up. It became a favourite and was a valuable meal in what were times of austerity.

Food really is an effective medicine with far greater healing properties than we have given it credit for.

Nettle soup recipe

Ingredients

A bag full of nettles with the leaves removed and washed

A couple of onions chopped. (I grow Welsh onions so I have them free all the year round. I simply wash and chop these up. Everything will be blended later.

Some potatoes or root vegetables (I use whatever is growing in the garden which may include Jerusalem artichokes, potatoes, carrots, burdock root).

Some wild garlic if it is available.

A couple of lovage leaves if available.

Some stock (I generally use bone broth made from a chicken carcase).

Method

Sweat the onions and garlic in a little butter for a few minutes.

Add the rest of the ingredients and simmer until all the ingredients are cooked. Blend serve and add a little yogurt

Pepper and salt are, of course, optional.

Other books by this author include:

- The EDS and Hypermobility Syndrome Diet
- Alleviating Symptoms of EDS
- Gastroparesis
- The EDS recipe book
- The Lipoedema Diet
- The Lymphoedema Diet: reverse and repair lymphatic damage
- The Anti-Virus Diet
- The Asthma Diet
- The Reluctant Bowel
- The MND Diet
- Why we live longer with higher cholesterol levels
- A dietary connection for MACS, POTS and EDS
- Identity: a self-exploration workbook *
- Journey Through Pneumonia

- Parkinson's Disease: dietary changes that work
- The Thyroid Diet
- https://www.amazon.co.uk/dp/B07TBHMV6N

*This book can be used alone or in small group work and is an excellent resource for those who are 'people helpers.'

Among many others

They are available on Amazon

Lynne has written a semi-autobiographical trilogy.

For the full range of books by this author, visit the author website on

https://www.amazon.co.uk/-/e/B07BPQZ5CD

https://www.amazon.com/-/e/B07BPQZ5CD

A percentage of the profits from the sale of these books go to support charities like the Exodus Project below.

The Exodus Project

My first introduction to the far reaching impact of The Exodus Project occurred when I was travelling around Cawthorne in one of their buses, visiting gardens. A young lad was happily munching on a sandwich. He looked up briefly, pointed to the driver and said,' He's my second dad, he is,' then he returned to his sandwich without further comment

Such remarks are often very telling and so I arranged to meet Jackie Peel and Martin Sawdon, at the charity's premises in Barnsley. They set up the Exodus Project 20 years ago. They moved into their current premises – a redundant Methodist church - in 2010.

Both Jackie and Martin have been youth workers in their church. Martin worked in housing for the homeless in addition to working in learning disabilities services in institutional settings.

The work that the Exodus Project undertakes is of paramount importance to the communities it serves. These were former mining communities which became disadvantaged after pit-closures. Currently about 400 children attend mid-week activities from Monday to Thursday inclusive. These activities include dance, drama, craft, music, sports and games. In addition, there are weekend camps, cycle treks, outward bound activities, bowling and swimming. The children are taught valuable life skills including how to cook and bake. It is all about teaching children how to fulfil their potential and learn skills they will be able to pass onto the next generation.

The grounds, once overgrown, have been turned into a play- and camping - ground. A miniature railway is in the process of being installed.

Martin and Jackie have developed a unique model in that The Exodus Project goes beyond dispensing services. They are keen to build up relationships with the whole family and not just the child that attends the mid- week clubs. In addition, once children have reached the age of fourteen, they are invited to help out with the younger groups as junior volunteers. Once they reach the age of eighteen, they become adult volunteers. This model provides a constant supply of help from individuals who have benefitted already from attending such groups.

The building is large and inviting. It is decorated with bold colours and has comfy seating. It is a real home from home; a haven for families who have been disadvantaged by the closure of the life force of its community.

Martin and Jackie have clear ideas about how they wish to develop the Exodus Project but the lottery funding which they benefitted from is no longer available. Sadly, they have had to close two of their clubs due to lack of funding. This decision wasn't taken lightly. They do have two charity shops which raises some money and they obtain some funding from outside organisations for the use of their facilities. However, this is clearly not enough to keep their clubs, weekend activities and building going to cater for the ever growing number of children who are benefitting from the work being undertaken here. Neither does it allow for future development.

Exodus do have a Just Giving page which can be found here if you wish to help further their work https://www.justgiving.com/exodus

In addition, you can keep up with activities on their Facebook page here

https://www.facebook.com/search/top/?q=the%20exodus%20project%20barnsley&epa=SEARCH_BOX

Recommended small businesses

https://skinkiss.org.uk/

https://favouritekafei.co.uk/?fbclid=IwAR1pW2OJNWCtFdIpgU7WWp9JQiQDxbBxu4GfzBfr6648snFYFERRYvGW7Ss

My Buy Me a Coffee website can be found here:

https://www.buymeacoffee.com/lynnedmnobl

The site contains a number of protocols as well as current health related topics

J.T. Parker

I. Introduction

Brief history of catfishing

The history of catfishing is long and storied, with evidence of people fishing for catfish dating back thousands of years. Native American tribes were known to catch catfish using various methods, including using spears, nets, and even bare hands.

Catfishing became increasingly popular in the United States during the 19th century, as European settlers began to discover the abundant catfish populations in rivers and streams. In the South, catfishing became a vital part of the local economy, with commercial catfishing operations developing along the Mississippi River and other major waterways.

In the early 20th century, recreational catfishing began to take off, as anglers discovered the thrill of catching these large and powerful fish. The development of new fishing equipment, such as rods, reels, and artificial lures, made it easier for people to target catfish and led to a surge in the popularity of catfishing.

Today, catfishing remains a beloved pastime for millions of anglers around the world. In the United States, catfish are the fourth most popular species targeted by recreational fishermen, behind only bass, panfish, and trout. Catfishing tournaments and derbies are held throughout the country, and catfish continue to be an important part of the commercial fishing industry.

The history of catfishing is a testament to the enduring appeal of these fascinating fish. Whether you are a seasoned angler or just starting out, there is always more to learn and discover about the world of catfishing.

Importance of freshwater catfish in the fishing industry

Freshwater catfish are a significant part of the fishing industry, both in the United States and around the world. These fish are highly valued for their meat, which is popular in many different types of cuisine, as well as for their size and fighting abilities. As a result, they are frequently targeted by both recreational and commercial fishermen.

One of the primary reasons that catfish are so important in the fishing industry is their abundance. Catfish can be found in many different bodies of freshwater, including lakes, rivers, and ponds. They are also relatively easy to catch compared to other types of fish, which makes them an attractive target for anglers of all skill levels.

Another reason that catfish are so important is their economic value. The catfish industry generates billions of dollars in revenue each year, including both commercial and recreational fishing. Many restaurants and food manufacturers rely on catfish as a source of protein, which helps to drive demand for these fish.

Catfish are also important from an ecological perspective. As bottom-dwelling fish, they play an important role in maintaining the health of aquatic ecosystems. They help to keep the water clean by consuming organic matter and other waste products, which can help to reduce the risk of harmful algal blooms and other types of water pollution.

In addition to their ecological importance, catfish are also culturally significant in many parts of the world. In the southern United States, for example, catfish are an important part of the local cuisine and have become a symbol of the region's culture and heritage.

The allure of catfishing

Catfishing is an activity that has captured the imagination of anglers worldwide. The thrill of hooking into a large catfish is something that cannot be easily replicated with any other species of fish. Part of what makes catfishing so alluring is the fact that these fish are not easy to catch, which makes it all the more satisfying when an angler finally lands one.

Another reason why catfishing is so popular is the wide variety of species that exist. There are over 3,000 species of catfish in the world, ranging from small, bottom-dwelling species to massive monsters that can reach over 600 pounds. This means that catfishing offers something for anglers of all skill levels and interests.

In addition to the challenge and variety, catfishing is also a great way to connect with nature. Many catfish species inhabit slow-moving rivers, shallow lakes, and other freshwater habitats, which are often located in beautiful, scenic areas. Spending time in nature is a great way to relax and recharge, and catfishing offers the perfect excuse to get away from the hustle and bustle of everyday life.

Furthermore, catfishing can be a social activity, whether you're fishing with friends or family. It's a great way to bond over a shared passion and to create lasting memories. Many anglers have fond memories of spending time on the water with loved ones, and catfishing is no exception.

Beyond the personal enjoyment and satisfaction that catfishing provides, it also has a significant cultural and historical significance. Catfishing has been an integral part of American culture since the days of the earliest settlers. Native Americans and early European settlers relied on catfish as a source of food, and as the sport of fishing developed, catfishing became a popular pastime. Today, catfishing is an important part of American fishing culture, and there are many festivals, events, and tournaments dedicated to celebrating this beloved species of fish.

II. Understanding Freshwater Catfish

Types of freshwater catfish

Freshwater catfish are a diverse group of fish found in a variety of water systems across the world. Like I mentioned in the last section: there are over 3,000 known species of catfish, with over 40 of those species found in North America alone. While all catfish share similar characteristics, such as their barbels and scaleless bodies, each species has its own unique features and characteristics that make them fascinating to anglers.

One of the most popular types of catfish for anglers is the channel catfish. These fish are found throughout North America and can grow up to 40 pounds in weight. They are known for their excellent fighting ability and their willingness to take a variety of baits, making them a favorite target for many catfish anglers.

Another popular species of catfish is the flathead catfish. These fish are known for their large, broad heads and their preference for live bait. Flatheads can grow up to 100 pounds in weight and are known to be elusive and challenging to catch, making them a prized catch for many experienced anglers.

Blue catfish are another popular species among catfish anglers. These fish are native to the Mississippi River and its tributaries, but have been introduced to other water systems across the United States. Blue catfish are known for their size, with some individuals reaching over 100 pounds in weight. They are also known for their excellent taste and are often targeted by both recreational and commercial fishermen.

Other species of catfish that are popular among anglers include the bullhead catfish, the white catfish, and the yellow bullhead. Each of these species has its own unique characteristics and behaviors that make them interesting to target.

Understanding the different types of catfish is important for anglers looking to target these fish. Each species has its own preferred habitat and feeding habits, which can help anglers determine the best tactics and techniques to use when fishing for catfish. With so many different species to choose from, catfish angling offers endless opportunities for anglers of all skill levels.

Physical characteristics and anatomy of freshwater catfish

Understanding the physical characteristics and anatomy of freshwater catfish is essential for any angler looking to catch this species. Catfish are well-known for their unique appearance, including their long whiskers and smooth, scaleless skin. There are several physical characteristics that distinguish different species of catfish, including their size, shape, coloration, and fin structure.

One of the most notable physical features of catfish is their barbels, which are long, whisker-like appendages that extend from their mouth. These barbels contain taste buds and sensory cells that help the catfish locate food in murky waters. Different species of catfish have different numbers and lengths of barbels, with some having as many as eight.

Catfish also have smooth, scaleless skin that can vary in color from dark brown to light gray or yellow. Some species have mottled or spotted patterns on their skin, while others have a more uniform coloration. Catfish have a broad, flat head and a long, tapered body that is ideal for swimming in slow-moving rivers and lakes.

The fins of catfish are also an important distinguishing feature. Most species have three dorsal fins, one adipose fin, and two or three pairs of pectoral fins. The pectoral fins are used for stability and maneuvering, while the dorsal and adipose fins provide additional support and balance. The caudal fin, or tail, is also an important feature for catfish, providing propulsion and steering.

Catfish are opportunistic feeders, and their anatomy reflects this. Their jaws are equipped with sharp teeth for catching and holding prey, and their digestive system is designed to process a wide variety of foods. They have a large stomach and a long, convoluted intestine, which allows them to extract nutrients from even the toughest prey.

In addition to their physical characteristics, catfish also have a unique anatomy that allows them to survive in low-oxygen environments. They have a specialized breathing system that allows them to extract oxygen from the water using their gills, as well as a secondary breathing organ called the swim bladder, which can function as a lung in oxygen-depleted waters.

Diet and habitat preferences of freshwater catfish

Freshwater catfish are known for their omnivorous diet, meaning they consume both plant and animal matter. Their diet can vary depending on the species and their habitat. In general, catfish are opportunistic feeders and will eat almost anything they can find. They often feed at night when it is dark, and they are less vulnerable to predators.

Some of the most common food sources for catfish include insects, crustaceans, mollusks, small fish, and even other catfish. In addition, catfish are known to scavenge for food, feeding on dead or decaying organic matter that falls to the bottom of the water.

When it comes to their habitat preferences, catfish are typically found in slow-moving or still bodies of water, such as lakes, ponds, and rivers with deep pools and slow currents. They are also known to live in areas with abundant cover, such as logs, rocks, and other structures, where they can hide from predators and ambush their prey.

The size and behavior of catfish also play a role in their preferred habitat. For example, larger catfish tend to live in deeper water where they can find larger prey, while smaller catfish may be found in shallower water with more vegetation and cover.

Another important aspect of catfish habitat is the presence of food sources. Catfish are known to follow their food sources and may move to different areas of a body of water depending on the availability of prey.

III. Gear and Tackle

Fishing rods, reels, and lines for catfishing

Fishing rods, reels, and lines are the most important pieces of gear for any angler, including catfish anglers. When it comes to catfishing, the type of rod, reel, and line you use will depend on the size and species of catfish you are targeting. In general, catfish are large and powerful fish that require heavy-duty gear. For rods, a medium to heavy power rod is recommended for catfishing. A rod with a fast or extra-fast action will also help with setting the hook and fighting large catfish. A length of 7 to 8 feet is ideal for casting and maneuvering in a boat. When it comes to reels, baitcasting reels are the most common choice among catfish anglers. They offer more control and power compared to spinning reels, which can be important when targeting larger catfish.

As for line, monofilament or braided lines are commonly used for catfishing. Monofilament lines are less expensive and easier to manage, while braided lines offer better strength and durability. A line with a test strength of 20 to 50 pounds is recommended for catfishing. It's also important to consider the leader material when setting up your line. A fluorocarbon or monofilament leader can help prevent the line from being cut by the catfish's sharp teeth.

Hooks, weights, and other terminal tackle

When it comes to catfishing, having the right hooks, weights, and other terminal tackle can make all the difference in whether or not you have a successful day on the water. There are a variety of options available, each with their own benefits and drawbacks.

Hooks are a crucial part of any angler's gear. For catfishing, circle hooks are a popular choice. They are designed to hook the fish in the corner of the mouth, making it easier to release them if you're practicing catch-and-release. J-hooks are also commonly used, but they are more likely to hook the fish deeper, which can make it harder to release them without causing harm. It's important to choose the right size hook based on the size of the fish you're targeting.

Weights are another important part of your terminal tackle. They help keep your bait on the bottom where catfish tend to feed. Egg sinkers, bank sinkers, and no-roll sinkers are all popular choices. Egg sinkers are a good choice when you want your bait to move with the current. Bank sinkers are designed to stay in place, making them a good choice when fishing in areas with a lot of current. No-roll sinkers are designed to stay in place, but their shape helps prevent them from getting stuck in rocks or other debris.

Other terminal tackle you may need include swivels, snaps, and leaders. Swivels are used to prevent line twist, which can cause your line to break. Snaps make it easier to change out your terminal tackle without having to retie your line. Leaders are used to prevent fish from biting through your line, and can be made of wire or fluorocarbon.

When choosing your terminal tackle, it's important to consider the size and strength of the fish you're targeting, as well as the type of water you'll be fishing in. You'll also want to make sure you have a variety of options on hand so you can adjust your rig based on the conditions you're facing.

In addition to choosing the right hooks, weights, and other terminal tackle, it's important to make sure your gear is in good condition. Check your line for any nicks or frays, and make sure your hooks are sharp. A dull hook can make it harder to hook the fish, which can result in missed opportunities.

Bait options for freshwater catfish

Bait is an essential element of catfishing, and the choice of bait can often determine the success of your fishing trip. There are numerous bait options available for freshwater catfish, and each has its own unique characteristics and advantages.

One of the most popular baits for catfishing is worms. They are readily available, easy to use, and inexpensive. They can be found in most bait and tackle shops or dug up from your backyard. Nightcrawlers, red wigglers, and earthworms are all effective for catching catfish.

Another popular bait is chicken liver. It has a strong odor that can attract catfish from long distances. Liver can be easily attached to a hook and casted out. Some anglers prefer to use livers that have been left out in the sun to age and develop a stronger scent.

Shrimp is another popular bait that catfish love. Fresh or frozen shrimp can be used, and they can be rigged onto a hook in a variety of ways. Shrimp can be used to target both small and large catfish.

Stinkbaits are a type of bait that are specifically designed to attract catfish. They come in a variety of flavors, including cheese, blood, and garlic. Stinkbaits can be purchased at most bait and tackle shops, or they can be made at home using a variety of ingredients.

Cut bait is another effective bait option for catfishing. It involves cutting up a piece of fish or other meat and attaching it to a hook. The scent of the cut bait can attract catfish from long distances, and it can be used to target both small and large catfish.

Live bait, such as minnows or crayfish, can also be used for catfishing. They can be rigged onto a hook using a variety of methods, and they can be effective for targeting both channel and flathead catfish.

Artificial baits can also be used for catfishing. Lures that imitate worms, crawfish, or other baitfish can be effective in certain situations. Anglers may choose to use artificial baits when live bait is not available or when they want to add some variety to their fishing trip.

When choosing bait for catfishing, it's important to consider the type of catfish you're targeting, the water conditions, and the time of year. It's also important to keep in mind that catfish have a strong sense of smell, so baits with strong odors are often more effective than those without. Experiment with different bait options to see what works best for you and the catfish in your area.

IV. Techniques and Strategies

Techniques for finding catfish

Finding catfish can be a challenge for anglers, but with the right techniques, it can be an enjoyable and rewarding experience. Catfish are bottom feeders and are often found in deep holes, channels, and other areas where the water is slow-moving. Here are some techniques for finding catfish:

1. Look for structure: Catfish tend to congregate near underwater structures such as logs, rocks, and brush piles. They use these structures as hiding places and to find food.
2. Use a fish finder: A fish finder can help you locate catfish by identifying underwater structures and changes in water temperature.
3. Pay attention to water temperature: Catfish prefer water temperatures between 70 and 80 degrees Fahrenheit. They will move to deeper water when the water temperature rises above 80 degrees.
4. Look for current: Catfish will often position themselves in areas where there is a current, such as near a dam or in a river channel.
5. Check out local hot spots: Talk to other anglers or do some research to find out

where the catfish are biting in your area. Look for areas with high catfish populations, such as lakes, rivers, and reservoirs.

6. Fish at night: Catfish are more active at night and will often feed near the surface when the sun goes down. Use a powerful light to attract catfish and use bait that will create a scent trail in the water.
7. Use scent attractants: Catfish have a keen sense of smell and are attracted to strong scents. Use bait that has a strong scent, such as chicken liver or stink bait, to attract catfish to your fishing spot.
8. Pay attention to weather patterns: Catfish tend to feed more aggressively before a storm and during periods of low pressure. Try fishing during these times for the best chance of catching catfish.
9. Experiment with different depths: Catfish can be found at a variety of depths, from just a few feet below the surface to over 50 feet deep. Try fishing at different depths to find where the catfish are biting.
10. Keep an eye on your fishing line: Catfish will often pick up bait and swim away slowly, so be sure to watch your fishing line closely. If you see the line start to move, reel in the slack and set the hook.

Popular methods for catching freshwater catfish

When it comes to catching freshwater catfish, there are several popular methods that anglers use. One of the most common techniques is known as bottom fishing. This involves using a weight to sink the bait to the bottom of the water, where catfish tend to feed. Anglers can use a variety of baits for bottom fishing, including live or dead baitfish, stink baits, and dough baits.

Another popular method for catching catfish is called drift fishing. This involves slowly drifting a baited hook or lure along the bottom of a body of water, allowing it to move with the current. This technique is particularly effective in rivers and streams where catfish often feed in the current.

Anglers can also use a technique called trolling to catch catfish. This involves pulling a baited lure behind a moving boat, typically at a slow speed. Trolling is a great way to cover a lot of water and locate active feeding areas.

Some anglers prefer to use a method called jug fishing, which involves suspending a baited line from a floating jug. This allows the bait to move freely with the current, which can be effective in areas with a strong current or in lakes with a lot of submerged vegetation.

Finally, some anglers use a technique called noodling to catch catfish. This involves reaching into underwater holes and crevices to grab the catfish by hand. This is a highly specialized and potentially dangerous technique that requires a lot of skill and experience.

Regardless of the method used, it's important for catfish anglers to be patient and persistent. Catfish can be finicky feeders, and it may take some time to locate active feeding areas. By using a variety of techniques and experimenting with different baits and lures, anglers can increase their chances of landing a trophy catfish.

Seasonal patterns and strategies for targeting catfish

Understanding the seasonal patterns of catfish behavior is critical to increasing your chances of catching a big one. Different strategies and techniques work best during different times of the year. During the summer months, catfish tend to move to deeper waters, especially during the heat of the day. This is when having a good sonar or fishfinder can come in handy. Look for drop-offs, underwater ledges, and other underwater structures where catfish may be hiding.

In the fall, catfish are more likely to be found in shallow water and close to the shore. This is because cooler water temperatures cause baitfish to move into shallower waters, which attracts catfish. The changing leaves and cooler weather also make this a great time to enjoy the outdoors while fishing.

Winter can be a challenging time to catch catfish, but it's not impossible. The key is to find deep water with good structure. Catfish become sluggish during the colder months, so fishing with live bait, such as worms or shad, may be more effective. Some anglers even use underwater lights to attract baitfish, which in turn attracts catfish.

Spring is when catfish start to become more active again, and feeding becomes a top priority. Look for areas with new growth and fresh vegetation, as this attracts baitfish and other prey. In the early spring, fishing with cut bait or chicken liver can be particularly effective. As the water warms up, switch to live bait or lures.

When targeting catfish, it's also important to pay attention to the time of day. Catfish are most active during low-light conditions, such as early morning or late evening. Night fishing can also be very effective, as catfish tend to be more active at night.

V. Fishing Regulations and Safety

Fishing regulations and licensing requirements

Fishing regulations and licensing requirements are an essential consideration for all catfish anglers. Fishing regulations vary depending on the state and location, and it is important to check the local regulations before heading out on a fishing trip. Most states require anglers to have a fishing license, which can be purchased online or in-person at various locations such as sporting goods stores, bait shops, and government offices.

It is important to note that fishing licenses are not transferable, and each angler must have their own license. Licenses are typically sold for specific time periods such as a day, week, month, or year, and fees vary depending on the duration and location. In some states, there may be additional requirements, such as a trout stamp or conservation stamp, which are needed to fish in certain areas or to keep certain species of fish.

Fishing regulations also include rules about the size and quantity of fish that can be caught and kept. Many states have size limits and bag limits for catfish, and it is important to follow these regulations to ensure the long-term health and sustainability of the catfish population. In addition, some states may have specific regulations regarding the use of certain types of bait or fishing methods, and it is important to be aware of and comply with these regulations as well.

Along with fishing regulations, catfish anglers should also be mindful of safety considerations. When fishing, it is important to wear appropriate clothing, such as a life jacket, and to be aware of potential hazards such as strong currents or underwater obstacles. It is also important to properly handle and release fish, especially if they are not being kept for consumption.

Conservation efforts are another important aspect of fishing regulations, as many species of fish, including catfish, are susceptible to overfishing. Anglers can help protect the catfish population by practicing catch-and-release, following size and bag limits, and reporting any illegal or suspicious activity. Additionally, many organizations and government agencies work to protect and manage catfish populations, and anglers can support these efforts by volunteering or donating to conservation programs.

Overall, fishing regulations and licensing requirements are important considerations for catfish anglers. By following these regulations, anglers can help ensure the long-term health and sustainability of the catfish population, while also enjoying a safe and rewarding fishing experience.

Safety considerations for catfishing

Catfishing can be a thrilling and rewarding experience, but it's important to keep safety in mind at all times. Before heading out on a fishing trip, it's essential to check the weather forecast and water conditions. Strong currents, high winds, and stormy weather can create hazardous situations, so it's best to stay on shore if conditions are unfavorable.

It's also important to wear appropriate clothing and gear. Comfortable, non-slip shoes or boots are necessary for walking on slippery rocks or banks, and a life jacket should always be worn when fishing from a boat. In addition, it's a good idea to bring a first-aid kit, insect repellent, and sunscreen.

When fishing from a boat, it's essential to follow all boating safety regulations and guidelines. Make sure that the boat is equipped with proper safety equipment, such as life jackets, a fire extinguisher, and flares. It's also important to have a reliable means of communication, such as a VHF radio or cell phone.

It's crucial to handle fish with care when catching and releasing catfish. Use a net to gently lift the fish out of the water, and avoid touching its gills or eyes. If the fish is to be kept, use a pair of pliers or a hook removal tool to safely remove the hook. Always handle the fish with wet hands, and release it gently back into the water.

When fishing in remote areas, it's important to let someone know where you will be and when you expect to return. In case of an emergency, it's crucial that someone knows where to look for you.

Lastly, it's essential to respect the environment and practice responsible fishing. Follow all fishing regulations and guidelines, and do not take more fish than you can consume or donate. Remember, conservation efforts are necessary to ensure the sustainability of catfish populations for future generations to enjoy.

Conservation efforts and the importance of catch-and-release

Conservation efforts and the importance of catch-and-release are becoming increasingly important in catfishing, as more anglers recognize the need to protect the populations of this species. Catfish are an important part of the ecosystem and play a vital role in maintaining the balance of aquatic life. They are also an important food source for many communities, making it all the more important to protect their populations.

Catch-and-release is a popular conservation practice among catfish anglers. This technique involves releasing the fish back into the water after it has been caught, allowing it to continue its natural life cycle. When releasing a catfish, it is important to handle the fish with care to minimize any harm that may be caused. A proper release will increase the chances of the fish surviving and returning to the population.

When practicing catch-and-release, it is important to use the proper equipment to minimize the stress on the fish. The use of circle hooks is one technique that can help reduce the chance of gut hooking, which can cause serious injury or even death to the fish. Using barbless hooks is another technique that can help make it easier to remove the hook from the fish, reducing the amount of handling time and stress.

It is also important to limit the amount of time the fish is out of the water. The longer a fish is out of the water, the greater the chance of harm occurring. When removing the hook, it is important to do so as quickly as possible and return the fish back into the water. It is also important to handle the fish with wet hands or gloves to avoid removing the protective slime coat on the fish's skin.

Catfish anglers should also be aware of the environmental impact of their activities. This includes not only catch-and-release, but also the use of bait and fishing techniques. The use of live bait, for example, can introduce invasive species into the water, which can have a negative impact on the ecosystem. Using artificial lures or cut bait can be a more environmentally-friendly option.

Another way to help conserve catfish populations is by following fishing regulations and licensing requirements. These regulations are in place to protect the population of catfish and ensure that they are not overfished. It is important to be aware of the rules and regulations in the area where you are fishing to avoid any negative impact on the population.

Finally, it is important to educate others about the importance of conservation efforts and the role that catfish play in the ecosystem. This can include teaching others about catch-and-release techniques and encouraging them to use environmentally-friendly practices when fishing. The more people that are aware of these issues, the greater the chance of protecting catfish populations for future generations.

VI. Preparing and Cooking Freshwater Catfish

Cleaning and filleting freshwater catfish

Cleaning and filleting freshwater catfish is an essential skill for any catfish angler who wants to enjoy a delicious meal of fresh fish. While some people might be intimidated by the process, it's actually quite simple once you get the hang of it. Here are the steps to follow:

First, you'll need to gather some tools. A sharp fillet knife, a cutting board, and a pair of pliers are all you'll need. If you want to make the process even easier, you can invest in an electric fillet knife.

Next, you'll need to prepare the fish. Remove any scales by running the dull side of a knife over the skin, working from the tail to the head. Then, cut off the head and tail of the fish.

Using your fillet knife, make a cut behind the gills of the fish and continue cutting down the length of the fish, following the backbone. Use the pliers to hold onto the skin and gently pull the fillet away from the bones.

Once you have both fillets removed, use your knife to remove any remaining bones. You can use a pair of needle-nose pliers or a fish bone tweezer to help with this process.

Finally, rinse the fillets with cold water to remove any remaining scales or bones, and pat them dry with a paper towel.

Popular recipes and dishes featuring catfish

Grilled Catfish with Lemon and Herbs

- Preheat grill to medium-high heat.
- Season catfish fillets with salt, pepper, and chopped herbs (such as thyme, rosemary, and parsley).
- Grill catfish for 4-5 minutes per side, or until cooked through.
- Serve with lemon wedges and a side of grilled vegetables.

Cajun Catfish with Rice and Beans

- Season catfish fillets with a Cajun seasoning blend (or make your own with paprika, cayenne pepper, garlic powder, and other spices).
- Heat a skillet over medium-high heat and add a drizzle of oil.
- Cook catfish fillets for 3-4 minutes per side, or until browned and cooked through.
- Serve with cooked rice and beans, and a side of hot sauce.

Catfish Po' Boys

- Mix together cornmeal, flour, and Cajun seasoning in a shallow dish.
- Dredge catfish fillets in the cornmeal mixture, shaking off excess.
- Heat oil in a deep skillet over medium-high heat.
- Fry catfish fillets for 2-3 minutes per side, or until crispy and golden brown.
- Serve on a hoagie roll with lettuce, tomato, and a drizzle of mayonnaise.

Baked Catfish with Tomatoes and Olives

- Preheat oven to 375°F.
- Season catfish fillets with salt, pepper, and paprika.
- Arrange fillets in a baking dish and top with sliced tomatoes and pitted Kalamata olives.
- Drizzle with olive oil and bake for 20-25 minutes, or until cooked through.
- Serve with a side of roasted potatoes or a simple salad.

Catfish Tacos with Cabbage Slaw

- Season catfish fillets with chili powder, cumin, and garlic powder.
- Heat oil in a skillet over medium-high heat.

- Cook catfish fillets for 2-3 minutes per side, or until browned and cooked through.
- Meanwhile, mix together shredded cabbage, chopped cilantro, lime juice, and a pinch of salt to make a slaw.
- Serve catfish in warm tortillas with the cabbage slaw and your favorite taco toppings.

VII. Catfishing Culture

The social aspect of catfishing

The social aspect of catfishing is an important part of the experience for many anglers. Catfishing can be a solitary pursuit, but it can also be a social activity that brings people together. Many anglers enjoy fishing with friends or family members and sharing the excitement of landing a big catfish.

Catfishing can also be a way to connect with other anglers and build a sense of community. Fishing clubs and organizations are a great way to meet other catfish anglers and share knowledge and tips. Social media has also made it easier than ever for anglers to connect with each other and share their experiences and photos.

Another aspect of the social side of catfishing is the tradition of passing down knowledge and skills from one generation to the next. Many catfish anglers learned to fish from their parents or grandparents and take pride in passing on their knowledge and techniques to their own children.

Catfishing can also be a way to connect with the local community. Many catfish tournaments and festivals are held in small towns and communities, bringing in visitors and boosting the local economy. These events often include food, music, and other entertainment, making them a fun way to spend a day with friends and family.

In addition to the social benefits, catfishing can also be a way to give back to the community. Many anglers participate in fishing derbies and other events to raise money for charity or to support conservation efforts. Catch-and-release fishing is another way that anglers can help to preserve catfish populations and ensure that future generations can enjoy the sport.

Stories and legends of catfishing

Catfishing has a long and storied history, and it has generated a number of fascinating stories and legends over the years. One of the most famous is the tale of the "kissing catfish," which dates back to the early 1800s. According to the legend, a group of men were fishing in the Mississippi River when they caught a large catfish. As they were preparing to kill the fish, one of the men noticed that it had a strange expression on its face, as if it were trying to communicate with them. The man decided to kiss the fish on the lips as a joke, and to everyone's surprise, the fish responded by kissing him back!

Another famous story involves the "blue catfish" of the Missouri River. According to legend, these fish are so large and powerful that they are capable of pulling boats upstream against the current. This may sound like an exaggeration, but there are plenty of fishermen who swear that it's true.

In addition to these stories, there are countless other tales of catfish that have been passed down through the generations. Some are funny, some are scary, and some are just plain strange. But all of them serve to illustrate the deep connection that people have with these fascinating fish.

Part of the appeal of catfishing is the mystery and uncertainty that surrounds it. You never know what you might catch, or what kind of adventure you might have. For some fishermen, this uncertainty is part of the thrill, and they are always eager to hear new stories and legends about the fish they love to pursue.

Of course, not all catfishing stories are about the fish themselves. Some of the most interesting stories involve the people who have pursued these fish over the years. From famous anglers like Zane Grey to local legends who have made a name for themselves on their home waters, there are countless stories of people who have dedicated their lives to catfishing.

The next time you're out on the water, take a moment to appreciate the stories and legends that have been woven into the fabric of catfishing. You never know what kind of inspiration or insight they might provide, and they are sure to add an extra dimension of excitement and adventure to your fishing trips.

Competitive catfishing and tournaments

Competitive catfishing and tournaments are a growing aspect of the sport of catfishing. These events bring together anglers from all over the country to compete for prizes and bragging rights. There are several different types of catfishing tournaments, including catch-and-release tournaments, live weigh-in tournaments, and online tournaments.

One of the most popular types of catfishing tournaments is the catch-and-release tournament. In these tournaments, anglers compete to catch the biggest catfish, but the fish are not killed. Instead, they are weighed and measured and then released back into the water unharmed. Catch-and-release tournaments are popular among anglers who want to protect the catfish population and promote sustainable fishing practices.

Another type of catfishing tournament is the live weigh-in tournament. In these events, anglers catch catfish and bring them to a weigh-in station, where they are weighed and then released back into the water. The angler who catches the biggest catfish wins the tournament. Live weigh-in tournaments are popular among anglers who want to compete for cash prizes and trophies.

Online catfishing tournaments are also becoming more popular. These events allow anglers to compete from anywhere in the world. Participants submit photos or videos of their catches, and the biggest fish wins the tournament. Online tournaments are a great option for anglers who may not be able to travel to a physical tournament location.

Competitive catfishing has become a major industry, with large cash prizes and sponsorships available for top anglers. The largest catfishing tournament in the world is the Catfish Conference Tournament, which takes place every year in Louisville, Kentucky. This tournament attracts thousands of anglers and fans from all over the world and offers large cash prizes for the top anglers.

In addition to traditional tournaments, there are also a number of catfishing competitions that are based on unique challenges or formats. For example, some tournaments require anglers to catch a certain number of catfish in a specific time frame, while others require them to catch fish of a certain size or weight.

Competitive catfishing is not just about winning prizes, however. These events also provide a sense of camaraderie and community among anglers. Participants often form close bonds with one another, sharing tips and techniques for catching catfish and supporting each other through the ups and downs of the tournament.

VIII. Resources for Catfish Anglers

Popular websites, forums, and social media groups for catfish anglers

In today's digital age, catfish anglers have access to a plethora of resources online to improve their skills, learn new techniques, and connect with other fishing enthusiasts. The internet has made it easier than ever before to access valuable information on catfishing. Here are some of the most popular websites, forums, and social media groups for catfish anglers.

One of the most popular catfishing websites is Catfish Edge, which offers a wealth of information on catfishing gear, techniques, and strategies. The website also features a blog section where anglers can read articles on various catfishing topics, such as how to catch big catfish, how to find catfish in rivers, and how to rig different types of baits.

Another great website for catfish anglers is CatfishNow, which offers a variety of articles and videos on catfishing. The website also features a forum section where anglers can connect with other catfish enthusiasts and share their tips, techniques, and experiences.

In addition to websites, social media platforms like Facebook and Instagram have become popular destinations for catfish anglers to connect and share their passion for fishing.

There are numerous Facebook groups dedicated to catfishing, such as "Catfish Anglers of America" and "Catfish Edge Community." These groups offer a platform for anglers to discuss different catfishing techniques and strategies, share their fishing photos and videos, and connect with other catfishing enthusiasts.

Instagram is also a great platform for catfish anglers to connect and share their fishing experiences. There are many popular Instagram accounts dedicated to catfishing, such as @catfishingofficial and @catfishingdaily, which offer a variety of catfishing content, including photos and videos of big catfish catches, tips and tricks for catching catfish, and gear reviews.

Another popular platform for catfish anglers is YouTube. Many catfishing enthusiasts have their own YouTube channels where they share their fishing experiences, techniques, and strategies. Some of the most popular catfishing YouTube channels include Catfish and Carp, Catfish Edge, and Catfish Dave.

In addition to these online resources, there are also numerous fishing forums and message boards where catfish anglers can connect and share their experiences. Some of the most popular forums for catfish anglers include Catfish1, Fishin.com, and Catfishing.net.

Recommended books, magazines, and other resources for learning more about catfishing

For catfish anglers who want to dive deeper into the world of catfishing, there are many resources available to help them learn more about the sport. From books to magazines to online resources, there is no shortage of information for those looking to improve their skills and knowledge.

One great book for catfish anglers is "Catfishing: Beyond the Basics" by Keith Sutton. This book covers a range of topics, from gear and tackle to specific techniques for catching catfish. It also includes information on different species of catfish and their behaviors, making it a great resource for anglers who want to understand their quarry better.

Another excellent book is "Catfish Hunter" by Bill Dance. This book covers everything from selecting the right gear to understanding different types of catfish and their habits. Dance also shares his personal experiences and insights into the sport, making it an engaging read for anglers of all levels.

For those who prefer magazines, "Catfish Now" is a great option. This magazine covers a range of topics, from gear and tackle to strategies for catching catfish in different conditions. It also includes articles on conservation and the importance of catch-and-release practices, making it a well-rounded resource for catfish anglers.

Another great resource is the Catfish Conference, an annual event that brings together catfish anglers, guides, and industry professionals from around the country. This conference includes seminars, workshops, and vendor booths, making it a great opportunity to learn more about catfishing and connect with other anglers.

Online resources are also plentiful for catfish anglers. The Catfish Edge website offers a range of articles, videos, and podcasts covering all aspects of catfishing. Another great online resource is the Catfish Angler Forum, a community of catfish anglers who share tips, advice, and stories about their experiences on the water.

Finally, for those who prefer video content, there are many catfishing channels on YouTube, such as Catfish and Carp, which offer a range of informative and entertaining videos on everything from gear and tackle to specific techniques for catching catfish.

IX. Conclusion

Reflection on the importance and enjoyment of catfishing

Catfishing is not just a hobby or a sport; it is a way of life for many people. It offers a unique experience that cannot be found in other forms of fishing. Catching catfish can be challenging and requires a certain level of skill, but it is also very rewarding.

Catfishing can be an important source of food for many people. Freshwater catfish is a delicious and nutritious fish that can be prepared in a variety of ways. For many anglers, catching catfish provides an opportunity to connect with nature and experience the thrill of the hunt.

Catfishing is also important for conservation efforts. Catch-and-release practices help to maintain healthy populations of catfish in the wild, while responsible fishing practices can help to prevent damage to the environment.

In addition to the practical benefits of catfishing, there is also a cultural significance attached to the sport. Stories and legends of catfishing have been passed down through generations, creating a rich history and culture around the sport.

Final tips and advice for catfish anglers

Now that you've learned about the different aspects of catfishing, it's time to put your knowledge to the test and hit the water. Here are some final tips and advice to keep in mind when catfishing:

1. Be patient: Catfishing requires patience and perseverance. It may take some time to locate the fish, but don't give up. Keep trying different techniques and baits until you find what works.
2. Use the right gear: Make sure you have the appropriate gear for the type of catfish you are targeting. Use a heavy-duty rod, reel, and line for larger catfish, and lighter gear for smaller catfish.
3. Keep your bait fresh: Fresh bait is essential when catfishing. Use live bait or fresh-cut bait and change it frequently to keep it fresh and attractive to the fish.
4. Pay attention to the weather: Catfish are more active in certain weather conditions. Overcast and rainy days are often the best times to fish for catfish.
5. Use scent: Catfish rely heavily on their sense of smell to locate food. Use scented baits or add attractants to your bait to increase your chances of success.
6. Keep safety in mind: Always wear a life jacket when fishing from a boat, and be

aware of your surroundings. Avoid fishing near dams or other hazardous areas.
7. Practice catch-and-release: Catfish are an important part of the ecosystem, and it's important to practice catch-and-release to ensure their sustainability. If you do keep fish for eating, only take what you need and follow local regulations.
8. Keep learning: Catfishing is a lifelong learning process. Keep learning about the fish and their behavior, and try new techniques and baits to improve your skills.
9. Enjoy the experience: Catfishing is not just about catching fish. It's also about enjoying the outdoors and spending time with friends and family. Take time to appreciate the experience and the beauty of nature.

The Freshwater Fisherman's Cookbook

Trout – Walleye – Perch – Pike – Bluegill – Catfish

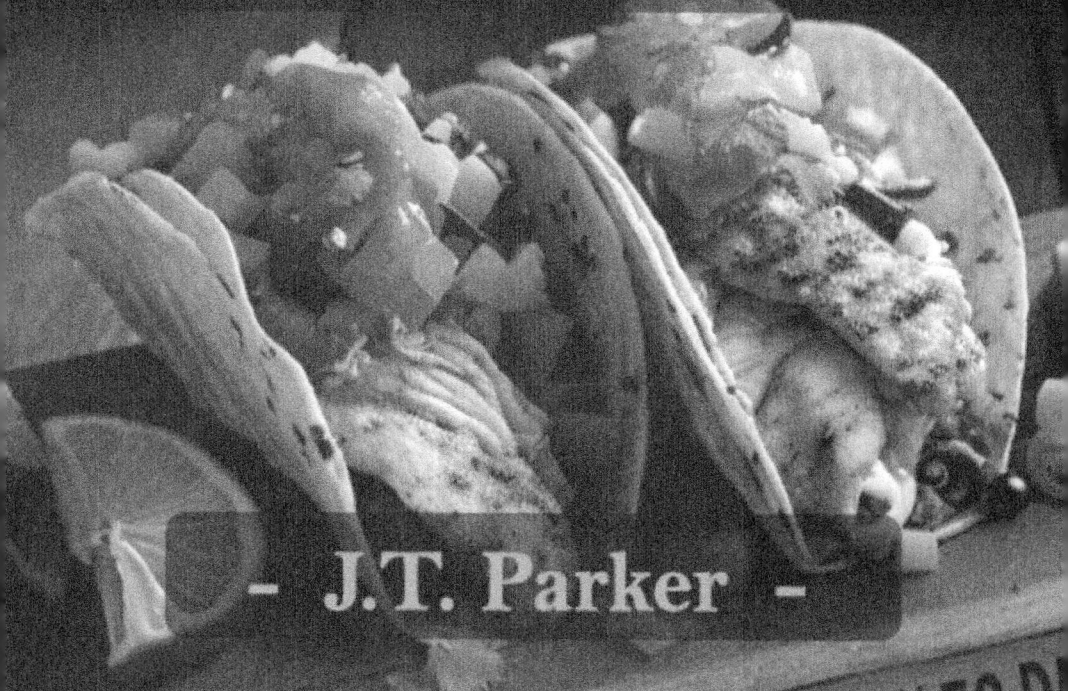

— J.T. Parker —

Printed in Great Britain
by Amazon